"As a son who experienced up close the painful yet precious course of Alzheimer's over two decades, I wish I had had the benefit of Dr. Post's book at hand. In this most enlightening study of the mystery of human dignity and identity under siege, he lifts the veil on that dreaded disease and provides insights, explanations, and hope for retaining the connections that count. Those unexpected, seemingly miraculous glimmers of the beloved as 'through a glass darkly' are here illumined both scientifically and spiritually as we confront our ultimate humanity—and human potential—face to face."   —Charles Scribner III, author of *Home by Another Route: A Journal of Art, Music, and Faith*

"Post brings to this book his tremendous compassion and understanding for the persons he calls 'deeply forgetful,' placing them on the same spectrum with all of us. The great humanity of his approach makes for a deeply rich, resilient, and nurturing community for us all. A must-read!"   —Gayatri Devi, MD, Director, New York Memory and Healthy Aging Services, author of *The Spectrum of Hope: An Optimistic and New Approach to Alzheimer's Disease and Other Dementias*

"I am pleased to see Dr. Stephen G. Post addressing themes such as consciousness and interconnectedness in his new book, which will contribute to the flourishing of humanity."   —The Dalai Lama

"The best summary of medical ethical issues in Alzheimer's disease from diagnosis to the end stage yet produced. Post is recognized worldwide as the foremost medical humanist and ethicist writing on this vitally important topic. This wonderfully written book awakens us to the continuing selfhood of these 'differently abled' people and helps us all to affirm their inalienable dignity." —Harold G. Koenig, MD, Director, Center for Spirituality, Theology, and Health, Duke University Medical Center

"Post magically connects the creative, the metaphysical, and the existential with practical ethics. His insightful analysis of human vulnerability, the fragile nature of our memories, the call for compassionate care, and the voice of the caregiver is grounded in consciousness."   —Sangeetha Menon, NIAS Consciousness Studies Programme, Indian Institute of Science

D1089452

"Stephen Post writes tenderly, lovingly, and wisely about those among us with failing mental faculties. This is a breakthrough book, innovative, humane, inclusive, and uniquely significant. Post thoughtfully probes every imaginable practical ethical question that a caregiver might have based on his three decades of ethics consultation with families. This is one book that every caregiver and professional should read." —Larry Dossey, MD, author of *One Mind: How Our Individual Mind is Part of a Greater Consciousness and Why It Matters*

"With story and solid intellectual grounding, this masterpiece is vital reading for the dementia field and far beyond." —Michael Splaine, Splaine Consulting / former Director, State Policy & Chapter Advocacy Program, Alzheimer's Association

"Dr. Stephen G. Post has greatly influenced Japanese care for deeply forgetful people, and he has inspired us to deliberate more about dignity, autonomy, identity, and authenticity." —Masako Minooka, MD, Executive Director, Japan Association for Clinical Ethics, author of *Ethics of Dementia Care in Japan*

"Dr. Stephen G. Post brings a hopeful and human perspective to those who think differently as they are living with cognitive changes while acknowledging the emotional and psychological impact on the family caregiver. His message and ethical approach to interactions support the enduring selfhood of the deeply forgetful, restoring dignity and honoring our shared humanity." —Jed A. Levine, President Emeritus, CaringKind, The Heart of Alzheimer's Caregiving

"In this serious and uplifting book we can feel Post's passion for the 'dignity of deeply forgetful people,' learn to notice and appreciate their expressions of continuing self-identity, and include them in our vision of a shared humanity. Drawing from years of experience, Post offers answers to the big ethical questions that Alzheimer's presents and challenges us all to set aside 'hypercognitive biases' and learn from these 'differently abled' people as we come to see them anew." —Joseph B. Martin, MD, Dean Emeritus, Harvard Medical School dignity for deeply forgetful people

DIGNITY
for deeply forgetful people

How Caregivers Can Meet the
Challenges of Alzheimer's Disease

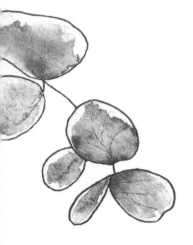

STEPHEN G. POST

with a Caregiver Resilience Program by
Rev. Dr. Jade C. Angelica

Johns Hopkins University Press
Baltimore

Note to the Reader: This book is not meant to substitute for medical care, and treatment should not be based solely on its contents. Instead, treatment must be developed in a dialogue between the affected individual and his or her physician. The book has been written to help with that dialogue.

© 2022 Johns Hopkins University Press
All rights reserved. Published 2022
Printed in the United States of America on acid-free paper
9 8 7 6 5 4 3 2 1

Johns Hopkins University Press
2715 North Charles Street
Baltimore, Maryland 21218–4363
www.press.jhu.edu

Library of Congress Cataloging-in-Publication Data

Names: Post, Stephen Garrard, 1951– author.
Title: Dignity for deeply forgetful people : how caregivers can meet the
    challenges of Alzheimer's disease / Stephen G. Post.
Description: Baltimore : Johns Hopkins University Press, 2021. | Includes
    bibliographical references and index.
Identifiers: LCCN 2021003212 | ISBN 9781421442495 (hardcover) | ISBN
    9781421442501 (paperback) | ISBN 9781421442518 (ebook)
Subjects: LCSH: Alzheimer's disease—Patients—Care. | Caregivers.
Classification: LCC RC523 .P668 2021 | DDC 616.8/311—dc23
LC record available at https://lccn.loc.gov/2021003212

A catalog record for this book is available from the British Library.

*Special discounts are available for bulk purchases of this book. For more
information, please contact Special Sales at specialsales@jh.edu.*

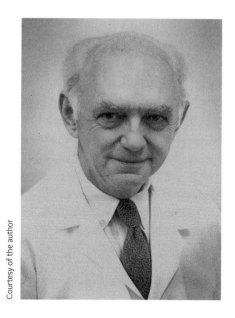

Courtesy of the author

Dr. Joseph M. Foley

1916–2012

This book is dedicated to Dr. Joseph Michael Foley, an outstanding clinical neurologist, educator, and academic leader who was noted for his kindness, his wonderful stories, and his gentle interest in every individual from whatever background or walk of life. Young Joe Foley was a standout at the Boston Latin School, received a full scholarship to the College of the Holy Cross, and went on to Harvard Medical School. He served as a navy medic in the Second World War, and he was awarded the US Bronze Star and the French Croix de Guerre for his actions to save others during the Utah Beach landing on D-Day. In 1961 he became director of the neurology division at Case Western Reserve University School of Medicine, where he stayed for the remainder of his illustrious career. He served as president of the American Academy of Neurology (1963–1965) and of the American Neurological Association (1974). He also chaired the first National Institutes of Health National Consensus Development Conference on Differential Diagnosis of Dementing Diseases (1986–1987).

In 1988, Dr. Foley recruited me from Fordham University-Marymount to Case Western Reserve University School of Medicine with the explicit challenge of developing a national program in medical ethics and the care of persons and families grappling with dementia. We worked together for two decades developing a clinical ethics consultation approach to caring for patients and their families, engaging them in countless "grassroots" dialogues so as to allow their voices to lead us. One of Cleveland's most beloved clinicians, he served tirelessly at the Joseph Foley Elder Health Center managing cases of Alzheimer's disease and other forms of dementia, improving the quality of lives and serving as one of the principal cofounders of the Alzheimer's Association at the national and local levels. Dr. Foley was the most influential person in my professional life and in the life of many others, including Joseph B. Martin, MD, who rose to become the renowned dean of Harvard Medical School some years after completing his residency under Dr. Foley at University Hospitals of Cleveland.

contents

[6] Respecting the Preferences of Deeply Forgetful People in Health Care and Research 173

with Phyllis Migdal, MD, MA

preface

This book is based on cases and themes not seen in my earlier work, *The Moral Challenge of Alzheimer Disease* (1995; 2nd edition 2000). In 2009 *The Moral Challenge* was selected as a "medical classic of the 20th century" by a distinguished panel of the *British Medical Journal,* which wrote: "Until this pioneering work was published in 1995 the ethical aspects of one of the most important illnesses of our ageing populations were a neglected topic." To be honest, things have not changed that much for the deeply forgetful and caregivers despite all the money invested in Alzheimer's pharmacology, which has been slightly effective at best, and only early on, primarily with regard to word-finding and attentiveness to tasks. There is no medicine to slow down the underlying progression of Alzheimer's, and caregivers eventually ask whether the treatments are worthwhile, especially when compared to the clear impact of music therapy or a service dog, which they can see and rejoice in as a loved one seems to come "alive inside," at least for a time.

I have grown older myself and more reflective, and thus while I remain unwilling to condone preemptive physician-assisted suicide (PPAS) for people with Alzheimer's who are newly diagnosed and still are able to act autonomously, I do not condemn it in these pages. I *do not* advocate for it because I see the lives of deeply forgetful people as worth living from beginning to end for all the reasons that are at the core of this book. Yet I have been reluctantly, and nonjudgmentally, present in informal pastoral support for a couple of individuals who, with family warmly at their sides, decided that they did not want to go on. Unable to convince them otherwise, I did the next best thing, which was to offer a respectful and appreciated presence, as I will describe in a chapter devoted to the topic.

All my writing is a tribute to Dr. Joseph M. Foley and to Alzheimer's Association chapters in every state across the country. It was Dr. Foley who encouraged me to do this work and who always displayed a gentle curiosity about my projects. In 1998 I became one of several people to have received the National Distinguished Service Award from the National Board of the Alzheimer's Association "in recognition of personal and professional outreach to the Alzheimer's Association Chapters on ethics issues important to people with Alzheimer's and their families." I don't value some awards, but this one I will always keep, and I owe it to having a mentor like Dr. Foley.

As for the basic structure of the book, I proceed from an introductory chapter to a chapter that takes up the theme of caregiver hope and where they can find it. Chapter three responds in a practical way to sixteen ethical issues that I have heard raised by thousands of caregivers, discussed with them in innumerable forums, and assisted in clinical consultations about. A fourth chapter takes up the question of "PPAS." Preemptive physician-assisted suicide for Alzheimer's disease is a question that will not go away. I try to handle such a hot-button issue in a fair-minded and nonjudgmental manner. Chapter five presents the core elements of the "ethics of respectful care" that caregivers aspire to. A sixth chapter focuses entirely on the extent to which we as caregivers can respect and abide by the previously or currently expressed preferences of a deeply forgetful person, especially with regard to clinical ethical choices. To bring this journey to closure, chapter seven connects back to chapter two and the theme of hope, and I respond somewhat pastorally to a question that has been asked of me many times: "Is Grandma still there?" This chapter builds from the well-documented experience of "terminal lucidity" that can occur in the days just before someone dies with dementia. I asked this question myself about my own grandmother, Grandma Post, years ago. At the time, I "felt" that she was still there underneath the communicative breakdowns, although she expressed her whole self sporadically. But I do not assert any kind of metaphysical position; the chapter is entirely factual.

These chapters are followed by a wonderful pastoral epilogue entitled "North Wind," written by a Chinese American caregiver and theologian who prefers to remain anonymous. And lastly, there is the all-important "Caregiver Resilience Program: Meeting Alzheimer's: Learning to Communicate and Connect," created by the ever-popular Rev. Dr. Jade C. Angelica, founder and director of Healing Moments for Alzheimer's (www.healingmoments.org).

DIGNITY
for deeply forgetful people

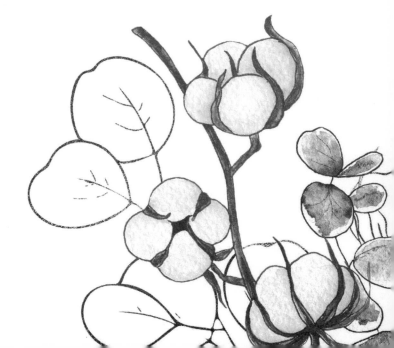

In Praise of Caregivers and Dignity

G ood caregivers are the salt of the earth—resilient, kind, and inspiring despite their many challenges. We celebrate the caregivers who in their labors of love bring light to a shadowy world. Even when inadequately supported, they prioritize the happiness and security of the deeply forgetful person they refuse to forget. Even when they have "spent down" into relative poverty, they often make their whole selves present no matter the task. There is much written about "the burden of caregiving," but caregivers also take intense joy in the sporadic expressions of continuing self-identity that rise up from beneath the surface of verbal chaos or protracted silence.

Caregivers also form a community of hopeful advocates, providing a counterweight to the "hypercognitive" (Post 1995b) and self-reliant cultural values that lead to disparaging descriptions of the deeply forgetful like "shell," "husk," "empty," "dead," and "gone." Words matter. At worst, a century ago the Nazis referred to deeply forgetful people as "life unworthy of life," or as "useless eaters," paving the way for the elimination of the "demented" through such notorious horrors as hypothermia experimentation (Post 2000). But the caregivers then and now stand defiant above such exclusionary values, beacons of dignity and grace. They are the ones who in each generous action or word sway the moral balance of the world and supply the living narrative of meaning that we most need.

Is there anything more ethically and spiritually uplifting in philosophy or theology than this simple vignette: A man makes daily visits to his deeply forgetful wife, who resides in a nursing home. He is asked by a friend why he does that, since she doesn't remember him. His simple reply is, "I remember her, which is what really matters, but she still smiles when I am there, and deep down she remembers."

Could there be a deeper expression of love than this email, written to me some years ago by a daughter soon after her father passed away:

Hello Dear Friends:

As many of you know, my father has been suffering from Alzheimer's disease for the past 4.5 years. It has been a long and often very hard road for him, for my mom, and for me too. However, as of 7 p.m. last night, my father no longer has to struggle with the disease that robbed him of every part of his being, except one. He never once stopped recognizing my mom and never, ever stopped reaching out to her and wanting to give her a kiss. No matter how many parts of his personality were lost, no matter how many hospital visits full of needles and catheters, no matter how many diapers, he always retained his kind, gentle sweetness and his European manners as a gentleman. In the end, things went very quickly for him. He simply closed his eyes and closed his mouth, indicating no more food or water.

How much deeply forgetful people benefit from gentle and respectful kindness! Should not all ethics begin with a thorough description of such kindness and care, rather than the abstract first principles conjured up in the past by philosophers who generally did not view caregiving as worthy of serious reflection?

———

Caregivers are to be praised because they do not doubt that someone who is deeply forgetful and cognitively compromised is worthy of moral inclusion in our human family and thus to be respected. Love pushes rationalism to the side, and the equality of inclusion based on consciousness itself comes into the moral foreground. Caregivers know that deeply forgetful people should never be dismissed on the basis of a relative diminishment of intellect (Post 1995b; Post 2000). Linear rationality and memory are only expressions of a much larger human consciousness, and someone who is deeply forgetful is as conscious of beautiful fall colors or exhilarating music as anyone else. *Equality of consciousness is more fundamental to moral standing than equality of intellect and memory.*

Whole human selves are so much more than sharp minds and keen memories. One of my colleagues, an epidemiologist who studies AIDS, tells the story of a young man with AIDS-related dementia who felt "written off" by his mentally agile friends. In response, he started a small business selling shirts to people with AIDS upon which was printed "Sum, I am." *Sum* is Latin for "I am," and he was trying to move beyond the philosopher Descartes's famous *Cogito, ergo sum,* Latin for "I think, therefore I am."

Deeply forgetful people should never be feared or devalued, bullied or derided. On the contrary, certain capacities such as kindness, mirth, and creativity may even be disinhibited from cultural constraints. Some years ago, while I was presenting at a conference in Bangalore at the Indian National Institute for Advanced Studies, the most famous Hindu philosopher in India endorsed my keynote by emphatically stating, "Correct, we must uphold equal regard and respect because the moral worth of a person is based on consciousness alone, not on memory or rationality. Namaste: we must honor the sacred consciousness within all people."

The Ultimate Reality of Human Interdependence

Caregiving is an active compassionate response to our interdependence with one another and with nature. We are all dependent when we come into this world, and for many months we cannot speak a word; we are all dependent in time of illness or injury, like when a fiercely independent adult child calls home in a panic because she has contracted a dangerous new virus. Most of us leave this life cared for by loved ones, friends, and the kindness of devoted professionals. *Dependence constitutes the deepest core of human experience, even when we pretend that we are self-made.* Our self-reliance is illusory because in fact we are each the beneficiaries of innumerable others who have cared for us in ways that helped make us who we are and sustained us. Forgotten in the busy workaday rush hour, someone (often a woman) is giving care back home with the children, in the school, in the hospital, in physical therapy, in hospice, in the nursing home, and just about everywhere. As our shared beliefs have withered, the bedrock truth remains that we are interdependent and relational beings who rely on one another no matter how much we may deny our fragility.

Seekers of Deeper Justice

Rev. Martin Luther King Jr. wrote often of "the love that seeks justice," and caregivers often become justice advocates. In any economically fair society, the reality of dependence and caregiving must be in the foreground of policy and economic support. Many caregivers in the United States are economically marginalized and reduced to poverty. This group represents a very large population if we consider all the dependent deeply forgetful people, children with developmental disabilities, and disabled people more broadly. Without acknowledging this obvious fact of dependence and attending to it, we cannot claim to have a just or flourishing society. It is right for caregivers and those they care for to receive something more than economic scraps.

Over the years I have heard countless stories from caregivers who felt that they were isolated, out of sight, and neglected with regard to both mental and physical health, often overwhelmed and unable to find the opportunity to get their own needs looked after clinically or otherwise. When they visit a clinic with their loved one and interact with physicians, nurses, other clinicians, and social workers, they indicate in surveys the good news that 90 percent of them feel listened to and communicated with clearly, but they also indicate the bad news that only 45 percent were asked if they needed help with caregiving or medical support themselves. Much more can be done to take better care of the caregivers. Nothing would help more than providing free respite care—having an outsider come into the home for a half day each week so that a caregiver can tend to their own needs. Many caregivers feel boxed in without help like this.

A deeper justice would begin with the ultimate reality of human interdependence and would help it work. Some years ago I attended an Alzheimer's Association National Public Policy Forum in Washington, DC, featuring the civil rights leader Congressman John Lewis and Alzheimer's Association leaders. Later in the day we marched to the offices of our senators and congresspersons, asking them to support the provision of subsidies to support just one half day of respite care for caregivers in need of a little time off. We were armed with the facts: one half day of respite per week would prevent the mental and physical stress on caregivers that can be so debilitating, and it would also save money—because refreshed caregivers can remain in their caregiver role considerably longer. The answer my team got from our elected congressional leader was negative, specifically: "No, if we did that for Alzheimer's caregivers, we would have to do it for other groups as well." A few months later an additional $200 million was appropriated to find a cure, but the cure for a disease this complex when we do not even know the cause to begin with has proven elusive.

Caregiving is so fundamental and so basic to human well-being and security that it must be at the core of any acceptable theory of justice or politics. But caregivers in cultures and politics of possessive individualism for the most part get only leftovers. Treating caregivers like this is wrong, because meeting caregiving needs is the very measure of a good and honorable society, consistent with human dignity, compassion, and love.

I emphasize the immense value of caregiving because there are to date no great scientific breakthroughs to eliminate Alzheimer's or most other diseases that cause dementia. These neurological conditions tend to be intractable, progressive, and slowly devastating. Maybe someday science will figure out how to prevent, delay onset, or cure Alzheimer's, but right now Alzheimer's has proven to be a very tough nut to crack. We hear researchers now talking about the "new approach" of attacking Alzheimer's even years before symptoms manifest, in the same way that we go after a tumor now as soon as the smallest cancer cells are detected. This approach makes sense. Nevertheless, there is more immediate hope in the social-environmental interventions of occupational therapists, innovative assisted living, music therapies, poetry readings, and even a dementia support dog than there is in any of the existing available drugs. Tender loving care, "music and memory," and kindness are the best treatments we have to date.

Learn First from the Caregiver

Over the years I have helped organize more than three hundred conferences for caregivers, often through the state or provincial Alzheimer's Association. At these events caregivers file in the door to learn whatever they can about how to care effectively, and the walls of the conference center are lined with tables from hospices, assisted living residences, and other entities including the local Alzheimer's service dog provider. These caregivers would then be seated in a hotel ballroom to listen to some well-intentioned neuroscientist download an hour of technospeak on the latest idea about a potential new drug pathway, or about the ever-questionable statistics on the positive effects of already-existing anti-dementia drugs. Over time this routine became so annoying to caregivers that they insisted conferences begin with a panel of speakers in this order:

1. A family caregiver who describes their experiences, ethical concerns, and wisdom gained across the chronological trajectory of Alzheimer's (usually diagnostic disclosure, advance directives, placing too much hope in magic-bullet medications when none exist, limitations on driving, nursing home placement, possibly stopping treatment for conditions such as diabetes and heart disease, end-of-life debates about the use of feeding PEGs and antibiotics, and so forth) (20 minutes)

2. An ethicist who has been in the trenches with these families to address these concerns (20 minutes)

3. A local physician who can address issues that arise (20 minutes)

4. An elder health attorney who encourages legal planning for medical decisions (15 minutes)

This panel discussion would be followed by an hour of lively and heartfelt questions and answers with the caregiver audience, many of whom shared their immense practical wisdom with one another in the process. Later in the day we would allow a full presentation on the latest science.

The present book is almost entirely shaped by these many conferences and events that began with the voices of the caregivers themselves, many but not all of whom were women.

Noticing Human Dignity

Dignity typically means something along the lines of "deserving respect." The word comes from the Latin base *dignitas*, which means "worthiness for honor and esteem." In the first sense of dignity, every human being has an intrinsic dignity that cannot be taken away, regardless of the extent of their forgetfulness. The second sense of dignity, which is dependent on a person's virtues and qualities, can be enhanced by awareness of a person's life story. A brief biographical sketch on the door of the person's nursing home room, as well as photos, meaningful objects, and playing their favorite music can help us recall someone's journey and who they are. Dignity always exists in both senses in deeply forgetful people.

The term "deeply forgetful people" is meant to help us notice the dignity of these people. They are not just "demented" or precipitously declined from a former mental state—which is the actual meaning of "dementia." "Dementia" is a word that is often used pejoratively to convey disapproval, disgust, dysfunction, and derision. Therefore, it is a term I use only sparingly throughout this book. It throws up a wall of separation between "them" and "us," and as the poet Robert Frost wrote, "Something there is that doesn't love a wall."

"Deeply Forgetful People"

"Deeply forgetful people" is a term suggesting that while those affected by dementia may struggle to remember and communicate, none of their limitations strip them of their personalities, various expressions of continuing insight into who they once were and still are, their tactile and food preferences, their often very remarkable artistic creativity, their emotions, their appreciation for the presence of others despite their forgetting names (as we all do), their consciousness of the world around them and its beauty, their astonishingly intense joy in the music with which they deeply identified earlier in their lives, their great comfort in the companionship of a dog, and of countless other manifestations of their whole selves. "We" are not really very different from "them," unless we choose to overvalue linear reason and independence at the expense of all the other human assets. "Deep forgetfulness" is a term that engaged me decades ago for its somewhat mystical intonations after an inspiring phone conversation with the philosopher Jamie Lindemann Nelson (Nelson and Nelson 1997).

If we stop overvaluing "hypercognitive values" (Post 1995b), we can start noticing and appreciating meaningful expressions of continuing self-identity at almost all levels of human interaction and self-expression in deeply forgetful people. When we take the time to notice we can begin to acknowledge that "they" are fully human persons after all, although they are further along on the continuum of human forgetfulness than most of us. *They are equal members of the human family deserving of every moral consideration.*

I provided respite for caregivers in Cleveland for many years. "Respite," as noted earlier, means taking over care, allowing caregivers to get away for shopping or any leisure activity, at least for a few hours. I was also leading many ethics workshops in Alzheimer's

Association chapters across the United States, Canada, and beyond with support from the National Institutes of Health and Association leadership, especially including the remarkable Alzheimer's grassroots organizer Michael Splaine.

While always saddened by the loss that progressive dementia brings to any victim while they are still insightful into their losses, I also took great joy in carefully observing the underlying continuities of self that allow for connectivity and relationship. I could see the heavy burdens of caregivers, but I could also see them smile intensely at those surprising moments of meaning when the underlying self-identity of a loved one becomes surprisingly manifest and coherently expressed. Thus, I began in the late 1990s to describe hope in caring for deeply forgetful people as "being open to surprises" (Post 2000).

Words of De-dignification

Recognizing the continuity between "them" and "us" constitutes the underlying moral challenge that caregivers rise to every day as they are close enough to notice in the details that their loved ones are still there and always maintain their dignity and worth no matter what. Caregivers stand strongly for deeply forgetful people, and they ask why disdain is too often directed at them. This is where caregivers exemplify Gandhi's dictum that love takes courage. Caregivers take firm exception to all the de-dignifying words and attitudes that exclude their loved ones from our shared humanity and often from adequate economic and social justice. Even in clinical settings I have sometimes heard a deeply forgetful person described using highly derogatory terms.

This linguistic de-dignifying exists because human beings sometimes build themselves up by diminishing the vulnerable. But it may also be that we somewhat more "intact" people go through the day with our own frustrating memory lapses, and down deep we are anxious about dementia as the dreaded condition we most hope to avoid. *Some people feel empowered and perhaps less anxious by de-dignifying deeply forgetful people, and thus the persistent dynamic of humiliation.*

But none of us are fully intact, and we all age. We might forget the name of a friend or student that we pass by when we should recall it with ease, and we are embarrassed because this lapse conveys a lack of care. Thus, we might say, "I am so sorry, but I am forgetting your name. Please remind me." This is pretty much how deeply forgetful people constantly feel before they reach a stage where they forget that they forget. We might forget where the car is parked and are grateful that at least we know it is out there somewhere to be found. We might walk away from a fresh cup of hot tea and open a cold bottle of water. Forgetfulness is basic to the natural human condition, and we spend a lot of time covering it up.

Connecting with Art and Music

By spending time with deeply forgetful people we can close the gap between "them" and "us" by seeing that we share many experiences in common. For example, people with Alzheimer's disease are generally capable of artistic creativity, just like we all are. They enjoy art programs, as demonstrated by innumerable art exhibits in memory care centers. The great Dutch American artist Willem de Kooning painted for thirteen of his final fourteen years with probable Alzheimer's. Later, his work, which he created while deeply forgetful, was exhibited at the Museum of Modern Art in New York. We need to see meaning and selfhood in "their" creative expression just as we do in our own. I knew a man who would come to art therapy class and draw very chaotic lines on paper, but there was always one line down the middle of the paper. I would ask him what that line was, but I could get no response. Finally, one afternoon he unexpectedly and loudly shouted out, "It's the old country road I loved to walk on." I could not know this man's consciousness, but maybe he was in some "flow" state of deep creativity, which people describe in terms of no longer being caught up in awareness of time, place, or ego.

Deeply forgetful people can find intense joy in music, as we all do. My colleague Jeffrey Trilling, MD, was for many years the chair of Family Medicine at Stony Brook School of Medicine. For five years he was in charge of a large unit for deeply forgetful people at the nearby Long Island Veterans Nursing Home. He once told me about the time he brought a Native American Lakota flute to work there one day, then sat quietly and played for a while. Gradually, nearly all of the forty or fifty people in the unit rose up and walked toward the sound, and he led them out onto the lovely green pasture adjacent to the unit. "None of them looked perplexed or anxious," said Jeff, "and I wondered to myself if they are closer to the Great Spirit than I have ever been." "Hypercognitive values" block some people from cherishing such beautiful moments. We are able to understand from our own experience what intense joy in music feels like, and this feeling can connect us with deeply forgetful people.

Deeply forgetful people have their culture and their dignity, but we have to notice those things, and we can only do that by being with them.

Three Cultures of Dignity

Returning to the reality of dependence and caregiving as the basic dynamic of human society, some cultures are better at affirming this primacy than others. It is instructive to reflect on how our culture tends to marginalize deeply forgetful people because of an emphasis on independence, rational autonomy, and economic productivity. We in modern Western cultures can perhaps better see the moral dignity and worth of deeply forgetful people by learning from other cultures.

The Confucian Approach in China and Japan

Among the Chinese, for instance, there is little interest in associating dementia in old age with disease. Instead, they prefer to think of it as natural; they accept the notion of a life cycle that concludes with a second childishness, and they are not fighting the same "war" the West is fighting against dementia with our attitude of fearful anxiety (Ikels 1998). Charlotte Ikels, my colleague when I taught at Case Western, would sometimes discuss this Chinese view in her classes on medical anthropology. Dementia for the Chinese culture is not so much dreaded as accepted. That culture is based on Confucian family values, the first and foremost being "filial piety." Secondly, it focuses on the honoring of familial structure and intergenerational reciprocity. Filial piety is a duty not undone by forgetfulness.

The Japanese culture is also much influenced by Confucian values, and by the concept of *amae*—defined by the renowned Japanese psychiatrist Takeo Doi in his classic book *The Anatomy of Dependence* (2014) as the ability "to depend and presume upon another's love" in trust and reciprocity. Because parents care for their utterly dependent infants, adult children feel the duty to return this "indulgence." Being dependent on another is not an embarrassment, as it might be viewed in the Western culture of individualism, but rather is considered a "pleasurable feeling." This also explains why in Japan individuals with Alzheimer's are typically treated with every life-extending medical technology available, although this practice is slowly changing, as I have discussed on two different visits to deliver plenary addresses for the Japanese Association for Clinical Ethics (Post 2014).

A renowned Japanese writer describes advanced dementia as a kind of spirituality, a means of release from anxiety over the future (Ariyoshi 1984). One thing I owe to the Japanese culture and four decades of marriage to my wife Mitsuko is this: I tend to find a quiet peace in being around deeply forgetful people, at least when they are not agitated and seem to be emotionally content. There are of course many very challenging moments that are anything but peaceful, as described in *The 36-Hour Day* (Mace and Rabins 2021). Perhaps a third of people with Alzheimer's have difficult emotional and behavioral challenges in the moderate stages, and caregivers require practical guidance and, hopefully, good professional assistance.

I once sat smiling for a quiet hour with a group of ten peaceful people with Alzheimer's on the porch of a temple in Kyoto with the Koshi Buddhist chimes wafting the calming sounds all around us and within us. I felt a certain "oneness" with them all. For those who wish to live a bit more in the "now," as the Buddhists put it, being around deeply forgetful people in a calm setting is not the worst thing imaginable—and much better than the loud Pachinko slot machine parlors a mile down the road.

But let us not in any way romanticize or spiritualize deep forgetfulness. Dementia is always a sad decline from a former mental state with huge economic costs. The Japanese are, of course, like everyone else, pursuing a magic-bullet treatment for Alzheimer's. In Japan life expectancy is about eighty-seven for women and eighty-one for men. With age alone being the major risk factor for Alzheimer's, about five million individuals in Japan are living with Alzheimer's dementia out of a total population of 127 million. Per capita, this is a much more challenging situation than in the United States, where about five million people have probable Alzheimer's out of a total population of 325 million. If we had the same life expectancy as the Japanese, we would likely have fifteen million affected individuals. We do need a magic bullet to end Alzheimer's disease, and science is doing its best to develop one with every new generation of devoted young researchers.

A third dignifying culture for deeply forgetful people is the African American one, which I address next in depth.

Love at Work in Poverty: Leo and Sister May

Isaiah 35 speaks of "the rose in the desert." Caregivers like May are that rose. May was dirt poor. I met her some years ago when a group of medical students accompanied me as I visited fifty homes of deeply forgetful African American people in the worst inner-city neighborhoods of Cleveland. One of the people I met was May's brother, Leo, who was eighty-two years old and had been diagnosed with probable Alzheimer's disease eight years before. He had been a professional boxer and a machine worker, and his body remained strong, although he was no longer able to forcefully push his caregivers away. Each day a health care aide visited, attending to the surgically implanted feeding tube and the catheter that emptied his bladder through an incision below the navel. The aide would turn Leo over, bathe him, and change his sheets, since he had recently become bedridden.

The firmness of his body contrasted with Leo's mental decline. That Leo was now bedridden was something of a relief to his caregiver sister May. Just a few months earlier, May had often been awakened by a breeze blowing through the door—Leo used to wander at night and sometimes managed to open the lock.

The house stank of urine from a huge guard dog that patrolled the first floor. The floorboards were of old beaten plywood, and the windows had been painted shut. There was no furniture downstairs except for an old sofa and a chair; upstairs there was only a shiny hospital bed with the medical fixtures needed for Leo's feeding tube and catheter. I felt that Leo was a captive to a strange combination of urban poverty and medically invasive technology. But when I questioned May, she stated that she'd never heard about the possibility of withdrawing treatment, or of doing assisted instead of tube feeding, nor had Leo when he still had his decisional capacities. "Wouldn't that be like killing?" May asked, when I sensitively raised the subject. I did not answer, but just listened. "Anyway, he don't do no harm," she added.

May was a wonderfully caring sister, but she was herself approaching eighty and was no longer very energetic. She had next to nothing. Caregivers can only care well when they are cared for. We cannot avoid the ways in which culture, ethnicity, economic class, and the injustice of marginalizing the needs of caregivers impact the care of deeply forgetful people. I respected May greatly, even though I struggled a bit with her keeping Leo in the grips of medical technology. I knew from one of her comments that she was probably collecting his social security or pension, and that was at least one little source of income in an environment of stark poverty. May was truly a victim, and she was right that there was no great harm in how Leo was being fed. And May was quite kind to Leo, who deserved her kindness.

Leo seemed to have adjusted emotionally to his condition and to be mostly free from pain, although he was anxious to be reminded of his identity. His speech had recently become more difficult to understand, so in what follows I have edited his words for the reader's benefit. At my initial visit, his first question was an unclear "Who am I?" May answered in a kind and jovial voice, "What do you mean? You know who you are. You're Leo. You were a boxer. You're my brother." Leo inquired, "Boxer? Was I?" "Yes, you were," responded May. "Where I am?" asked Leo. "In Cleveland, where you've been living for years," said May. "Mobile?" inquired Leo. "No, you were born in Mobile, but now you're in Cleveland," May told him. "Who am I?" repeated Leo. "What, you forgot again who you are? You're Leo, silly," May responded. "School, school. Who was my mama?" Leo asked. "Why, you silly bones," answered May, "you know your mama was Leona, and she was my mama too, and you don't go to school." "Who am I?" Leo asked again.

I was impressed by May's constant kindness, and I saw her as a good role model for life in general.

The cycle of questions, answers, and forgetting went on, and throughout I could see that however deeply forgetful he might be, Leo was still there underneath his difficulties. There was still a Leo in that room, and he was not "gone" or "absent," let alone "already dead"—words sometimes used in our hypercognitive culture that prevent us from taking note of all the interesting ways in which Leo and May were still deeply connected.

As the conversation between brother and sister continued, I began to see that Leo quite enjoyed asking May these questions. There was no obvious frustration on his part when he repeated something he had just asked a minute ago, because every word was new. May's patience and kind voice seemed to relieve any anxiety on his part. She did simple but meaningful things, like touching his hand or patting his shoulder. So in this dilapidated old home I saw love at work, and I knew that deeply forgetful people matter ethically, spiritually, and socially just as much as any members of our human family.

Deeply forgetful people express emotion and respond to kindness; they respond to their environment with pleasure or fear; most carry on conversations of a sort; and they can be treated in a manner that diminishes the moments of terror that must accompany their sense of self-fragmentation. Simple expressions of reassurance do much good; and May had a tone of voice that also clearly soothed Leo. Thus, there are numerous ways to provide meaningful care that can make the experience of dementia less frightening and inhumane.

An Ethics of Care

The way to begin an ethics of dementia is not with moral abstractions but with listening attentively to caregivers and affected persons in their homes, or as they participate in support groups and share their experiences. This is an ethics of care (Kittay 2019) grounded in concrete experience and meaningful solidarity. The ethics here begins with an appreciation for the deeply forgetful person's well-being and a willingness to engage their remaining capacities and memory; it can be discovered only in practice and dialogue; it must be practical rather than abstract.

When we approach them in this way, we see that deeply forgetful people have strengths—for example, they often can remember how to perform tasks they did earlier in life, tasks that may give them a sense of fulfillment. A man suffering severe dementia still remembered his boyhood chore of carrying wood, and walking with a bit of kindling in his hand dramatically improved his self-esteem and emotional state. Behaviors that appear meaningless may not be so: the person who wanders may actually be searching for something or someone; and realizing this fact makes appropriate responses possible. Environments can be designed to provide appropriate visual, tactile, auditory, and physical stimulation without causing sensory overload and consequent distress, and cues can be built into the interior design of nursing homes to help residents find their way around without feeling lost. Such designs are intended to protect residents while maximizing ambulatory opportunities and independence.

THREE TIPS FROM MAY

1. Something can always be done for deeply forgetful people in the form of love and respect. May was truly present with Leo, and she did not grow sharp or impatient, even when she was pressing him a bit on his forgetfulness. She felt that she was just trying to reconnect him somewhat with the world and his life narrative, and she saw this as adding to his dignity. To some degree she was correct, although at a certain point attempts like those become counterproductive and even agitating as dementia progresses. There was a time, and I saw some of this with my grandmother, when "senile" people would be seated in a lecture hall to listen to some "reality therapist" tell them the date, the year, and the name of the president. We now recognize that entering the world as the deeply forgetful person defines it is the most peaceful solution after the disease progresses past a certain point.

2. May responded to Leo's understandable feelings and needs, even if he was struggling to express them. She saw him as a whole self, and not just cognitively. She identified and responded to those feelings and needs, and she had a gentle curiosity about what he was trying to utter.

3. May knew her emotional and physical limits, as every caregiver must, so she had steady respite caregivers coming in to substitute for her twice a week. She said that this respite is what kept her sane and kind.

Caregiver Questions as Alzheimer's Unfolds

My experience with May and Leo confirmed that Alzheimer's disease presents many big ethical questions. In addition to the huge problem of bias against the lives of these differently abled people, a complete study of ethical and social issues in dementia must include the following:

- Diagnostic truth-telling
- Implementation of advance directives
- Debates around preemptive physician-assisted suicide
- Limitations on freedom in the interest of safety
- Research ethics
- Use of the relatively ineffective anti-dementia drugs
- Restrictions on driving
- Physical and pharmaceutical restraints
- Achieving a just balance between family and social obligations in meeting the costs of long-term care
- The basis and limits of filial duties
- Sexual intimacy
- The problem of pain
- The moral significance of quality versus quantity of life
- Communication techniques
- Overtreatment and discomfort involved in efforts to extend life
- The use of dubiously effective artificial nutrition and hydration
- A good dying within a hospice-like model

These are just a few of the questions and issues that arise as one follows the chronological course of the illness experience that I have been writing about over three decades. Perhaps the biggest question of them all is this (it is also included in the list above): Should we allow preemptive physician-assisted suicide for those who are so inclined, not because they are imminently dying, but precisely because they may have many years ahead of them and do not wish to endure this journey?

2

Hope in Caring for Deeply Forgetful People

Why It Matters and Where to Find It

Hopelessness is a destructive emotional state that can overwhelm caregivers, thereby diminishing their well-being and health; it can then adversely affect the quality of care those caregivers provide. Maintaining hope is perhaps the most essential strength of the caregiver, who somehow carries on and even flourishes despite real daily challenges. Hope has to do with our readiness to see the dignity that is always there despite deep forgetfulness and behavioral difficulties.

Over the years I have studied hope and optimism in women, drawing on the data from the Women's Health Initiative. We have, for example, found that hostility and hopelessness contribute over time to chronic heart disease in women. This result would be expected given what we know about vascular disease and protracted or chronic stress caused by emotions such as hostility, rumination, and despair (Salmoirago-Blotcher et al. 2019). Many caregivers are themselves older adults, so of great relevance is the 2020 study done by the Harvard T. H. Chan School of Public Health that analyzed the Health and Retirement Study data set (N = 12,998, mean age = 66 years). That study found that after controlling for all variables, a greater sense of hope was associated with better physical health and health behavior outcomes (reduced risk of all-cause mortality, fewer chronic conditions, lower risk of cancer, and fewer sleep problems); higher psychological well-being (increased positive affect, life satisfaction, and purpose in life); lower psychological distress; and better social well-being (Long et al. 2020).

Clearly hope is a vital asset for the caregiver. How can the caregiver maintain hope, especially when it is so easy to spiral downward into anger and hostility without it? Hope is not Pollyannaish optimism—the idea that a positive outcome is inevitable. Hope is more of a realistic motivation toward the goal of providing good care, and it involves activity, a can-do attitude, and a belief that there is a path to a better future (Groopman 2005).

Where can a caregiver find and build hope? We can begin with the powerful story of Orien Reid, who navigates hope in a way that many African Americans do, given their historical faith community, although various other major sources of hope will be considered too.

Hope in Faith: Caregiver Orien Reid

Some call Alzheimer's a living funeral—a devastating event when the person you love, the keeper of all your childhood stories, precious memories that can only be shared between the two of you— like those of a husband and wife, brother and sister, aunt and uncle, or parent and child—is lost in the myriad of plaques and tangles of Alzheimer's disease. It steals much more than memories—it ravages everyone it touches; but what it doesn't kill is the immutable, indestructible love—the one force that drives caregivers to give so much physical and emotional energy to a loved one with Alzheimer's.

Nothing replaces the human touch, the human spirit, and human love. Alzheimer's can't destroy those things, the very things that caregivers give in the twenty-four-hour/seven-days-a-week experience that's driven by their love. They are truly doing the work of the angels.

Orien Reid, a friend of Rev. Martin Luther King Jr., raised on the Morehouse College campus, and the finest chair of the national Alzheimer's Association that I have ever known, wrote me the following narrative:

My family has had a lot of experience in caregiving, because four members of my family have been struck by Alzheimer's. My grandmother was first—they called it senility when I was growing up. She was demented most of my life and died in 1962 when I was sixteen years old. I watched as my mother and her closest sister cared for my grandmother. Then twenty-six years later it was my turn, when my mother was diagnosed with Alzheimer's. She died in 1992. Three years later, my uncle J.D., her brother, began the slow descent into Alzheimer's. He died in 1997. Just two years before Uncle J.D. died, my aunt Vernetta, the same one who cared for my grandmother, the same one who dutifully called my mother every week during the course of her disease, discovered that Alzheimer's was her destiny too. My cousin Brenda is literally giving her life in caring for my aunt.

The one quality that resonates through each one of us living the caregiving experience is a strong sense of commitment, bonding, and love. There was never a time in my life when I didn't feel my mother's absolute unconditional love. She was an elegant, intellectually talented, very articulate and gutsy Southern lady. A beautiful steel magnolia— soft outside, but tough as nails. When I was just six months old, she left my father, who was pastoring a church in Topeka, Kansas. She moved with me to Atlanta and found a job at Morehouse College as secretary to the legendary president, Dr. Benjamin Elijah Mays. Dr. Mays was affectionately known as "Buck Bennie," because he stood tall, bucking racism at every turn. He was a great leader, motivator, and mentor to so many. The South was a hotbed of segregation and intimidation. But Dr. Mays inspired and encouraged students, faculty, and staff like my mother

to stand tall in the face of adversity: "It is not your environment, it is you—the quality of your mind, the integrity of your soul, the determination of your will—that will decide your future and shape your life."
An ordained Baptist minister and former dean of Howard University's School of Religion, Dr. Mays had an inner spirituality. His love of students, love of equality, and, yes, his true altruism made him an admired spiritual mentor. Indeed, it was his thoughtfulness that led him to offer to have his wife take care of me while my mother attended faculty-staff meetings. Mrs. Mays, a beautiful woman, was nurturing and fun. She would let me comb her hair and always had a surprise for me in her cupboard.

It was Dr. Mays's help and support that enabled my mother to develop her civic leadership. We lived on the Morehouse campus all of my life. That setting, while intellectually stimulating, also provided some degree of protection when my mother held civil rights rallies on the steps of the Georgia Capitol. She was a woman who stood up for what she believed, even meeting with the governors of the state and yes . . . a woman who found herself, in what should have been a peaceful retirement, retreating into a very confusing, disorienting world of Alzheimer's.

The diagnosis was the most painful blow in my life. You see, as an only child, I had grown up as the center of my mother's life. She was a doting, loving, and nurturing mother who protected me. I remember at six years old, having an attack of acute appendicitis. I remember she cried while preparing me to go into surgery. She kept saying she wished she could take the pain away from me because she didn't want to see me suffer. Ironically, as a caregiver, I felt the same way about her. I wanted to protect her, to save her from this terrible disease.

That's what motivates so many caregivers. Of course, there is also a feeling of loss of the parent, spouse, or loved one you've grown to cherish. But it's much more than that. It's also that you don't want to see them suffer, and you wish you had the power to stop the pain they're enduring. That is unconditional love.

The physical and emotional cost of the earnest unconditional love and protection that caregivers give day after day and hour after hour can't be measured in dollars and cents. The caregiver is often called the second or hidden victim of Alzheimer's. The majority of caregivers are women, and a survey done for the Alzheimer's Association found the average caregiver spends sixty-nine hours a week caring for someone with Alzheimer's.

Let's use my cousin for example. She's a well-educated woman with a master's degree in counseling. She has taken care of my aunt for eight years. There's little doubt of her commitment. Like many caregivers, she loves her mother and wants to take care of her, but the stress of caregiving has forced her to take a non-professional job with meager wages. She's told me she needs "a job where she doesn't have to think." It's a catch-22 because she is underemployed and suffering from caregiver burnout. But she can't see any other viable solution.

A month ago, my aunt fell. My cousin said when she took her to the emergency room, the physician asked, "Which one is the patient?" He finally convinced her that she couldn't do this anymore. My aunt was admitted to the hospital and then released to a nursing home.

Today, my cousin browbeats herself because the care in the nursing home isn't as good as what she could do for her at home. It's taken every bit of energy I could muster to convince her that her health is also at risk. She has chest pains and shortness of breath, and she has delayed her own follow-up treatment because she's concerned about taking care of her mother. She cooks meals for my aunt and carries them to the nursing home after a full day at work. She has plunged into a depression, and misses her mother terribly, even though she is exhausted herself.

The research tells us what's happening to my cousin happens so frequently to caregivers. The studies say that 80 percent of those caring for someone with Alzheimer's disease suffer from not only high levels of stress but also depression. Listen to these words from Lynn Halevic, caregiver of her husband:

He is near and yet so far.
I feel his warmth, but not his strength.
I need his strength so badly
My stress is at times breaking me.
I try to understand, but I fear I'm failing.
I need my best friend.
Where has my love gone?
The spills, the dirty Depends, the laundry.
They all attack my spirit.
They attack me emotionally and physically.
I cry, and I scream a silent scream.
I long to break the silence,
But the scream sticks in my throat.
My love, where has it gone?
Why have I lost it?
I want to find it again.
I want my champion, my strength back.
He is gone.
My love is gone.

It is the pain of this experience and the love for my mother that drove me to find an outlet for my grief. It's the kind of hurt that never goes away. I remember asking God not why this happened to me, but why her? I couldn't think of any conceivable positive outcome of this experience—not for my mother, nor for me.

But if you really do believe that, as my dad used to say, "God gives man free will," and we make the choice of how to use the experiences we have, then you understand why some of us make difficult choices and choose to fight instead of surrender.

And I firmly believe that no matter what the problem is, if I ask, as I do each day, for divine guidance, that indeed that's what helps me get through each day. Divine guidance helped me survive the caregiving experience. Divine guidance and the many experiences of watching my mother, Dr. Mays, and indeed, Dr. Martin Luther King Jr. and others *fight for what they believed, gave me the courage to give up a successful twenty-six-year career in television, to become a volunteer chair of the national board of the Alzheimer's Association out of a sheer drive and belief that this was my way of fighting this disease.*

And I believe that even today it is both my mother's love and my love for her that continue to drive me. As a chair of the Association, there were many frustrating, difficult times, but I was always clear why I would never throw in the towel. I didn't when I took care of my mother, and I won't start now. Everything I do today, all that I have ever achieved and will ever achieve is because of the love, guidance, and strength of both of my parents. They were exceptional people, and I have a legacy—a legacy of love that will never die. I leave you with these final thoughts from a devoted caregiver:

EVERY MOMENT

He eats, and I feel comfort.
He laughs and I feel joy.
He speaks and the sound of his voice
Frees something inside me
That soars up to the heavens
Proclaiming a bond
That can never be broken

Every moment together
Is a treasure that I lock
Safely away in memory.
I am a dam bursting,
Unable to contain the fullness
Of my love for him.

Religiosity indicators (such as "prayer, comfort from religion, self-rated religiosity, and attendance at religious services") are especially significant as coping resources for African American women caregivers (Picot et al. 1997). Spirituality is a clear stress deterrent, and therefore also impacts depression rates, which are extraordinarily high in those caring for individuals with dementia. These authors suggest that if religiosity indicators are shown to enhance a caregiver's perceived rewards, health care professionals could encourage caregivers to turn to their religiosity to reduce the negative consequences and increase the rewards of caregiving.

There are many caregivers for whom hope cannot be fully discussed outside of a spiritual or religious tradition. Whether it is in the form of the Roman goddess Spes (hope) or the Pauline affirmation of "faith, hope, and love," hope evokes the spiritual in many cultures, for hope is so important to our lives that it is considered sacred. It is fair to say that a caregiver who has no hope cannot long survive. Inscribed in stone above the gate to Hell in Dante's *The Divine Comedy* are the words "Abandon all hope ye who enter here" (Canto III, line 9). Without hope, caregiving can only be a "burden," but with hope it is both a burden and, at times, a joy.

Hope in the Biomedical Model

So much investment is devoted to finding biomedical solutions to prevent or cure Alzheimer's, and someday the miracle cure may indeed come to be. This is everyone's hope. But three decades have passed without a preventive or curative drug. We can now look for more ways to enhance quality of life with the help of the arts, an expansion of music and memory interventions, as well as other ways to connect deeply forgetful people with their self-identity. Hope lies in a sense of connectedness with people who have Alzheimer's—and a feeling for their quiet dignity. In fact, economic resources for training and interventions that improve the quality of life for people with Alzheimer's need to be equal to the resources dedicated to biomedical solutions. This kind of support will allow every caregiver to have a strong sense of active agency in which they can do their jobs properly.

Persons with Alzheimer's and their families greet the emergence of new compounds to mitigate the symptoms of dementia with great hope but with too much expectation. These compounds, among which are the cholinesterase inhibitors, slightly elevate the amount of acetylcholine in the brain, providing a small boost to communication between brain cells. In the earlier stages of the disease, while enough brain cells are still functional, these drugs can in some cases slightly improve word-finding, and maybe attentiveness to tasks, for a brief period in the range of six months to possibly two years in rare cases. Thus, some symptoms can be slightly mitigated for a brief period of time, but these drugs have no impact on the underlying course of the disease, and none reverse or cure Alzheimer's. Some affected individuals, after taking any new compound, whether artificial or natural, may exude a burst of renewed self-confidence. Occasionally people with an early diagnosis of Alzheimer's report a mental clarity, as though "a fog has lifted," but only for a brief period at best, and then that clarity fades. By analogy, we treat a brain tumor with aspirin, which can be slightly helpful for some patients for a few symptoms for a while, but clearly aspirin has no impact whatsoever on the growth of the tumor itself.

In defense of the biomedical physicians prescribing various new drugs as they come along, this is what they are trained to do. Drugs are more beneficial in treating behavioral issues, but they are not as beneficial in treating dementia itself; this syndrome remains intractable and irreversible. It is hard for medical professionals to know how to respond to the caregiver's passion for the possible. Should unrealistic caregiver hopes be indulged by drug prescription for emotional reasons? There is nothing clearly wrong with prescribing anti-dementia drugs in response to caregiver hope, although the money expended for new compounds of relatively marginal efficacy could be spent more effectively on environmental and relational opportunities. Clinicians may or may not caution both persons with Alzheimer's and their caregivers against viewing a drug as a miracle cure. Nevertheless, reports of a "fog lifting" are interesting anecdotally and sometimes euphoric at the start. This is partly due to the placebo effect, of course. Medication needs to be placed within a full program of dementia care (including emotional, relational, and environmental interventions) so as not to be excessively relied on; family members should be respected when they desire to stop medication; even when medication is desired, families need to appreciate the limits of current compounds.

There will certainly be something new down the road that will surpass by far anything we currently have available. Gains may be incremental while science continues to take steps in the liberation from deep forgetfulness that we all seek for ourselves and for the future. But for caregivers this hope for a new drug is a passive kind of hope. Hope rises and falls and rises and falls, because it is dependent on news of a breakthrough in some lab and then on some pharmaceutical company that decides to take a gamble. The fluctuations in such passive hope result from the fact that the caregiver is not an active participant in the process, but rather simply waiting. We should of course hope for a new and more effective treatment for memory loss, but that hope should not replace the active kind of hope that motivates us to roll up our sleeves and make a difference.

––––––

Healthy aging is a good idea for us all, especially those with an increased risk of Alzheimer's. A combination of the proper diet, weight management, regular exercise, and stress management can help. Perhaps diet will become particularly important, especially for those with a family history of Alzheimer's—explicitly, those who have two first-degree relatives (parent or sibling) with the condition are at increased lifetime risk.

Those with a family history might wish to believe that a Mediterranean-type diet may help prevent dementia (Scarmeas et al. 2009), but this is hard to prove. And yet, in a study, 2,148 subjects in upper Manhattan, sixty-five years or older, with a median age of seventy-eight years at baseline, were followed for four years. Of this group, 253 were diagnosed with "probable Alzheimer's." Seven different dietary patterns were examined. After adjustment for demographic factors, body mass index, caloric intake, and genetic risk, only one pattern—the Mediterranean diet—was associated with lower levels of Alzheimer's: a whopping 38 percent reduction in a four-year period. Vascular health is clearly important in staying healthy and cognitively intact. Maybe the Greeks had it right twenty-three centuries ago in that old Hippocratic passage about dietary measures: "I will apply dietetic measures for the benefit of the sick according to my ability and judgment; I will keep them from harm and injustice." In other words, we should look to diet, exercise, cognitive stimulation, pro-social activities, reduced stress, and perhaps the midlife use of certain medications or natural substances that may be preventive.

Hope in Being Open to Surprises

The idea of hope as "being open to surprises" is a definition I developed over years of listening to caregivers for the deeply forgetful in support groups and community dialogues across every state in the country, every province in Canada, and in ten other countries from

Scotland to Japan. Despite even major memory losses, there are always sporadic indicators of continuing self-identity that emerge and that reveal the loved one who still exists beneath the everyday silence or chaos. These moments of insight into intact selfhood can actually be very revealing—and of lasting significance—once we learn how to understand what is being communicated. From these revelations meaning arises for the caregiver, who more fully understands that to be deeply forgetful and with little awareness of time and place by no means implies that a loved one is merely a "shell" or a "husk."

Every caregiver must have abiding hope that their kindness and their compassionate actions make all the difference in the life of a loved one. Hope is deeper than optimism; optimism is to hope as happiness is to joy. Optimism is more or less an established genetic set point, although it can be affected by one's social-relational context. It is mostly a dispositional trait and may sometimes feel inappropriate. Hope, in contrast, is a fine-honed virtue arrived at through enduring at least some hardship. Martin Luther King Jr. could speak of hope running down the mountains like a river, but the word "optimism" would not have fit the bill. I once asked an African American pastor what he thought about hope, and his response was, "It is something that we have had to specialize in, because we have suffered so much as a people." Hope is shaped and formed over time. It is deeply realistic about the facts and foresees clearly the struggles likely to come; optimism is rather superficially chipper without really acknowledging future struggles, and thus it has a certain avoidant quality and can be fleeting. Optimism can crash, while hope is resilient in the hard times when suffering is close to overwhelming and caregivers have to dig deep. Caregivers must determine to be hopeful despite all, and they must make this decision again and again. They have every right to hope even against hope. Whereas happiness is dispositional and usually quite dependent on external circumstances, joy is considered a virtue, both deeper and more stable than happiness.

Caregivers become the best "noticers," the people who perceive and respond to the details that others fail to pick up. Hope is about noticing and responding to the inner person that endures underneath the chaos. In this sense, hope is an activity and assertion of agency, rather than something passive, as in "I hope that someday they come up with a better pill for memory loss." "They" have not done so yet, at least not one that makes any real difference, though they might claim otherwise. Meanwhile, hope must come from cultivating a sense of community—and from noticing.

So how does a caregiver sustain hope? By noticing that contrary to the negative depictions of the deeply forgetful as "just a husk," "already dead," and so on, they are investing their minds and hearts in a loved one who is still there. Most caregivers are familiar with Dan Cohen's Music and Memory interventions (www.musicand memory.org), and with his documentary *Alive Inside.* When a deeply forgetful person is brought back in a fuller realization of self-identity through connecting with favorite music from earlier in life, they sometimes will be able to respond to a few carefully crafted questions afterward. While such experiences are fleeting for the affected individual, for caregivers these experiences are not fleeting at all. Suddenly, they are able to see that grandma really is still there—they just did not know how to connect with that inner being.

Hope in Man's Best Friend:
The Alzheimer's Service Dog

Not everyone loves dogs, of course, so service dogs are not for everyone. But if your loved one ever had a favorite dog earlier in life the

Alzheimer's service dog is often a great idea, so try it out. As a matter of justice, for example, why not provide every caregiver and deeply forgetful person who wants one with a well-trained "dementia dog"? Many people with dementia find intense joy and love in having a loyal, unconditionally loving dog, and caregivers can look on with a smile. Imagine the delight experienced by a deeply forgetful person able to sit with a well-trained dog in her lap, smiling, stroking the dog's fur, and remembering times gone by in a relaxed and peaceful state of mind. I served as a member of the advisory board of the Alzheimer's Center at the University of Stirling in Scotland in the 1990s when the research on the immense benefits of trained support dogs was being studied. The positive result that research offered is a worldwide phenomenon nowadays, and I am pleased to have been supportive. Now everyone with dementia in Scotland, Australia, and other countries has access to a wonderful companion dog if they desire one. Dogs do not care if an older adult is deeply forgetful, and when well-trained they can be extremely helpful with ambulation, relational warmth, and loyalty. There is no currently available drug that does anything like as much good as a support dog—and a dog has no side effects.

A caregiver, Meryl Berdugo, approached me after I gave a plenary session in a Brooklyn Heights conference on programs around the world that allow deeply forgetful people to have the benefit of trained guide dogs. She wrote me an email the next day:

> *Bringing Lola to see Alzheimer's patients has made a tremendous differ-*
> *ence in helping me open up the line of communication. Take Marvin,*
> *who is ninety-one and lives at home with his wife. He has advanced*
> *Alzheimer's. He has a full-time aide and sleeps in his own room while*
> *his wife has the master bedroom. Marvin had walked into her bedroom*
> *and fell asleep in the bed since the morning. . . . The aide and his wife*
> *couldn't get him up. I walked in the room with Lola, put her paws up on*

him and said, "Marvin get up, look who came to visit." Marvin popped
up, excited to see Lola. I was able to lure him out of bed and into the
family room, where his wife was. He couldn't contain his excitement.
His wife and the aide couldn't believe it. Lola brought back his memory
of his dog Sparky!

I have been elated to track case after case where trained dogs are making a huge difference in the quality of life of deeply forgetful people and making things easier for their caregivers as well. How much intense joy they bring to most people with Alzheimer's, allowing them to brighten up and connect in a manner that brings security, peace, and a smile. Dogs are always a part of "The Eden Alternative" settings in nursing homes, along with plants, birds, and so forth. Labrador seems to be the preferred breed. For any caregiver interested, the best website on Alzheimer's and dogs is www.dogs4 dementia.com.au, which explains: "Dogs 4 Dementia is the first time in Australia that expert Dementia Centre consultants have partnered up with skilled Assistance Dogs Australia trainers to place dogs into the homes of people living with dementia. A dog is carefully chosen to match household personalities and trained to meet their specific needs." The right dog will generally do more to give a deeply forgetful person a good life in which they experience warmth and joy than pretty much any other intervention known to humanity at this time, although personalized music is exceptionally helpful too. But that kind dog is there around the clock bringing affection and relationship and working synergistically with the needy caregiver whose burdens are thereby somewhat alleviated.

Is there any medication yet that can do anything close to this?

How do you get a service dog for a deeply forgetful person? In the United States we need to train more dementia service dogs, but any caregiver can search the internet and find a trainer.

Of course, a caregiver needs to look after a dementia service dog, but deeply forgetful people often like to help out when they are able. Dogs can do a lot of things, but to mention a few:

NINE WAYS A DOG CAN HELP

· Pick up dropped items.

· Open and close doors.

· Provide stimulating tactile companionship.

· Keep the handler from getting lost or wandering.

· Trigger an alarm for emergency situations.

· Remind a person that it is time to take a pill (through an electronic sound in a medicine bag).

· Make a deeply forgetful person happy.

· Take the emotional pressure off a caregiver and make their lives a little easier and more joyful.

· Be completely loyal to a deeply forgetful person and be a source of accepting love.

Hope in Twelve Aspects of the Enduring Self

Over years of interactions with deeply forgetful people, I have not met one individual who did not express aspects of continuing self-identity at least sporadically. The abstract philosophical idea of total disconnection between the then "intact self" and the now "no self" is thus contrary to observed fact (Post 1995a). Moreover, this mistaken idea contributes to a loss of both meaning and hope in caregivers as well as to potential mistreatment and abuse of deeply forgetful people, for it denies the narrative of a life as experienced over time.

Psychologist Steven Sabat has described meaningful interactions with individuals who are far advanced in the progression of dementia, demonstrating that many actions, emotions, and utterances have meanings that we fail to detect (Sabat 1994, 2001; Sabat and Cagigas 1997). For example, a deeply forgetful person who is agitated and crying might seem to be engaging in chaotic meaningless emotion and behavior. But place the individual's cherished symbolic object in their hands, like the baseball cap that they identified with all their adult life, and they will immediately calm down and smile.

Deeply forgetful people may not have linear rationality in terms of projecting goals and operationalizing them, but they do have symbolic rationality all the way through the illness experience, and they can connect with objects of special meaning just like they can connect with deeply learned music from earlier in their lives. We assume that their behavior is inexplicable when in fact they may well be conveying something meaningful, if only we could understand.

THE TWELVE ASPECTS

There are at least twelve aspects of the enduring self under conditions of deep forgetfulness, and probably more. They include the self as:

- Creative
- Symbolic
- Emotional
- Relational
- Somatic
- Musical
- Rhythmic
- Aesthetic
- Olfactory
- Spiritual
- Tactile
- Cognitive

Let me highlight some of these aspects of the enduring self by describing a few brief case histories, a couple of which appear to involve the mysterious phenomenon just before death known now as "terminal lucidity," a topic discussed in depth in chapter seven.

CASE ONE. I met Mr. G. in 1988 in a nursing home in Chardon, Ohio. After reading a brief sketch about his life, I sat down to talk with him, and started out by asking him how his sons were doing. Although he could not understand or respond, he placed a twig in my hands and gave me a huge warm smile. Then he surprised me by uttering the words "God is love." I thanked him and then gave the twig back. Afterward, I asked the nurse to tell me about the twig. She said that when Mr. G. was a boy growing up as a Christian on an Ohio farm, he loved his father very much. Every morning, his father gave the boy the chore of bringing in kindling for the fireplace. Mr. G. had retreated back in time to his boyhood, to a period of fatherly love that provided an emotional safe haven. The twig was a profound symbol of the love Mr. G. felt as a boy from his dad. So I learned from Mr. G. that even when the present is a buzzing chaos, a person with deep forgetfulness can find tranquility in recollections of the past, and from that safe haven can remind us of his or her enduring selfhood (Post 2007).

Of course, this nurse might have seen the twig as just some object that Mr. G. had latched on to for no reason at all; she might then have taken it away from him as an annoyance. This might well have caused Mr. G. to melt down in an emotional crisis requiring sedation. But the nurse understood something about who Mr. G. was, and how much this twig meant to him. Perhaps she had discussed this with his sons, who visited regularly.

CASE TWO. Memories in the Making is a nationwide program that explores whether people with dementia can reveal themselves through art. Many artists from around the United States now volunteer to lead these programs in most major cities and towns. What we have discovered is that even in the most advanced stages of dementia, individuals will express remnants of self-identity. They may not be able to communicate by speech or proceed from point A to point B over time. True, they live to a considerable degree in the pure present, but we need to be very careful not to assume that the connective glue between present and past is ever completely gone. Sometimes, such assumptions evaporate when we allow these people opportunities to express their self-identity through the re-creation of a symbol. In October 2006, the *Columbia Daily Tribune* (Missouri) ran a story I told the reporter about a man with dementia who clung to his cowboy hat until the very end of his life, even bathing and sleeping with it. It turned out that he had worked in the steel factories of Cleveland and had always dressed in a country-and-western style. He knew his identity was somehow connected with that cowboy hat, or so stated his daughter, Sharen Eckert, president of the Cleveland Alzheimer's Association at the time. The article also included an anecdote from Debra Brook, local director of the Alzheimer's Association in Columbia, who told of one elderly person with dementia who did not recognize his daughter any longer. "When the man joined the Memories in the Making program, he worked for weeks drawing a series of horizontal and diagonal lines on paper. He was not conversant and had not been for months. Although generally unresponsive when asked what he was drawing, one morning after a good night's rest he suddenly blurted out, 'Directions to my daughter's house.'" Despite his decline, this gentleman was still expressing love for his daughter through creativity.

CASE THREE. Dr. Joseph Foley died in June 2012 in Cleveland at the age of ninety-six. A distinguished neurologist, Joe had always had a fabulous sense of humor and regaled his friends and colleagues with hilarious stories; over twenty years this Bostonian son of Irish immigrants taught me over a hundred Irish jokes. At my last visit with Joe, the day before he passed on, Joe was quite forgetful, though he had no formal diagnosis of dementia of which I was aware. He was unable to converse. So I started telling him some of the old Irish jokes that he had taught me over the years:

"So Joe, what's the Irish definition of hospitality?" No response.

"It's makin' someone feel perfectly at home while you be a wishin' they were." And Joe broke out in laughter.

I learned that someone can be unable to communicate but if properly stimulated their mirthful nature can manifest even very near the end of life. Underneath the communication problems there was still a glorious jovial Irishman.

CASE FOUR. In March of 2013, I visited the Long Island Veterans Nursing Home and spent some morning hours in the facility for veterans with severe dementia. About thirty vets filled an activities room. As far as I could observe, almost none of them were conversant or responsive when they were called by name, and most had that thousand-miles-away empty stare. Then came the big moment, when the activities director started the music. Strains of "New York, New York" and "That's Amore" floated out across the room, and about two-thirds of these old-timers started to sing along with the voices of Frank Sinatra and Dean Martin as the words appeared on the big screen. Then came "You're a Grand Old Flag," and it seemed like the singing got louder. A few more vets chimed in, and soon five of them were standing up, saluting the flag. I felt like I was witnessing a miracle. Deeply embedded and remembered music, including hymns, with which individuals identify autobiographically, touches their enduring selves at a profound and hidden level, eliciting a renewed sense of who they are. Immediately after this music session, in the space of just a few brief minutes, four of the six vets we approached with a simple closed-ended question—"Hello, [first name], do you love America?"—responded with statements like "Sure do," or "You bet." Some went on to share even longer comments. It was as though they had arisen from a deep slumber.

Research indicates that the medial prefrontal cortex (just behind the forehead) links memory, music, and emotion. This appears to be one of the last parts of the brain to atrophy in the progression of Alzheimer's disease (Janata 2009). For more information about a major care movement called Music and Memory, see www.musicand memory.org.

CASE FIVE. For my grandmother, the manners and etiquette she knew from her childhood were always readily apparent, even at the end of her life. In fact, out of the blue she would still correct me: "Stevie, please do not put your peas on your fork with your thumb." "Yes, Grandma Post, I will be careful about that," I would respond, as I had when I was a child, many years earlier. She had gone back to a time in our relationship that was comforting to her and joyful, and I wanted to come along with her. She was still there, but had gone back to a happy time.

CASE SIX. Olivia Hoblitzelle (2008), author of *Ten Thousand Joys & Ten Thousand Sorrows: A Couple's Journey through Alzheimer's*, emailed me a few days after we shared a panel together at the Times Center in Manhattan for the New York Alzheimer's Association's Charles Evans Lecture. Olivia had read something of mine, and wrote, "It reminded me of a moment with my beloved mother, a poet, author, and something of a philosopher. In that late stage when words are gone except for those very occasional moments, she looked at me intently and said forcefully, 'God, physics and the cosmos.'"

I wondered where this statement from Olivia's mother came from. The phenomenon of terminal lucidity is quite well documented in cases of Alzheimer's disease. An individual may be virtually mute but somehow in those final hours some clarity returns. Where does this clarity come from? What does it mean? No one has pondered this phenomenon more than the distinguished Harvard neurologist Dr. Rudy Tanzi. In his YouTube presentation, "Unexplained end-of-life lucidity in dementia patients," Tanzi talks about people just before they die recalling events and conversing with loved ones. He cannot explain this phenomenon, and thinks that perhaps in the future science will begin to grasp it.

CASE SEVEN. Another example of terminal lucidity is described in an email I received in 2016 from Cathy Chapin, a caregiver in Canada:

> *I spent three hours yesterday afternoon with my sister and I tried to make sure that every facial expression, the tone of my voice, the intentionality of my focus was positive and loving. I didn't understand a word she said but it didn't matter. I felt love by being loving and Wendy felt love by receiving my love. At the end of our visit she said, "I want you to stay with me always."*

CASE EIGHT. A Stony Brook University medical student wrote this reflection about his grandfather as his mother described his last moments of surprising lucidity:

> *It was in his last moments that my mother seemed to be rewarded for all her hard work. My grandfather looked at my mother and spoke to her with complete lucidity for the first time in a year. He talked about the old times when he used to walk her to school. Then he talked about me and told her to make sure I kept working hard in school. And the last thing he said was how proud he was of her and that he loved her. The next morning he was gone.*

In these cases and countless others like them we see or hear moments of real clarity and surprising evidence of continuing self-identity.

We cannot explain this. We have no model. But these cases are all evidence that underneath the communicative chaos or the haunting silence, deeply forgetful people are proclaiming, *I'm still here* or *This is what I want to be remembered for.* Our challenge as caregivers is to stimulate the more salient of the aspects of continuing self-identity in any given individual.

The jaded and the skeptical among us may doubt the significance of these hints, labeling them the last insignificant residues of deteriorating brain matter. But for most people around the globe, and followers of spiritual traditions of all sorts, these hints are more than that. Hindu friends in Gambier, Ohio, for example, have another interpretation. Dr. Sangutha and team are all professional caregivers at a nearby facility. Dr. Foley and I took them to lunch one day and asked them why they put so much effort into caring for so many patients with dementia, many of whom were older and had the dual diagnosis of Alzheimer's and Down's. They replied that each human being carries within a small particle of divine mind, or as their faith expresses it, *atman (soul) equals Brahman (God).* Perhaps the individual mind is more mysterious than we often assume and is not merely an epiphenomenon of matter. In all my years working with families I have never contradicted a caregiver who perceives the outlines of an eternal soul beneath the veil of his or her loved one's day-to-day communicative disabilities.

If we take the time to be present, we can observe an enduring self in the deeply forgetful. Therefore, let us learn to pay careful attention to, and find meaning in, expressions and behaviors that often have more communicative significance than we might at first realize. Let us respect—from the Latin *respectare* ("to re-look" or look deeper)—the enduring self those expressions and behaviors reveal. In doing so, we might find greater purpose and meaning in our task as caregivers as a result.

As I have suggested above, a person with dementia is not as "gone" as we might suppose, and caregivers who are truly present all report surprising interactions that the biomedical model tends not to emphasize with its "stage theories" of neurological decline. In fact, variation and heterogeneity break through these models of decline, even though it is possible to speak of a general progression. Every case, of course, is different, and the right social, psychological, and environmental prompts can reveal the self that these theories tend to diminish. There are those moments, often early in the morning after having slept well, when a person with severe dementia surprises us with a meaningful word, a moment of recognition. Again, such moments complicate overly concrete theories of staged progression. A person incapable of conversation may join with others in singing a verse of a deeply loved song. These glimmers of a fuller presence merit our respect, as caregivers and as fellow humans. Therefore, sit down, make eye contact, and call that person by name as if expecting an answer—even though it may not come today. This action is more than symbolic. It is how we affirm the enduring self. Our task is always one of affirmation and connection.

But what blinds us to the signs of the enduring self? What makes some prefer to see the glass as half-empty rather than as half-full? Why do we hear pejorative terms used to describe the deeply forgetful? Here I believe we must confront various biases and prejudices, many of which have their roots in hypercognitive values.

Hope in the Moments of Joy

Carol Bowlby Sifton of Canada, a leader in caregiving based on her experience and teaching, has reflected on caring for her father thus:

We can choose to lament, to be lost and lonely, or we can choose
to seek out the joy in what we do and let it renew our resolve.
Sometimes joy finds us. It may take the form of a fleeting look of
recognition and warm embrace from the loved one with dementia. It may take the form of shared laughter from a silly mistake,
shared words from a familiar prayer, or shared lyrics from an old
song sung just off key. Sometimes joy is present but we are too
busy to recognize it. (Sifton 2004)

*One learns in caring for deeply forgetful people that it is better to be always
kind than always right, as is true of life in general.* There is no need to
correct deeply forgetful people after a certain point of adjustment to
their condition by trying to bring them back into temporal reality by,
for example, reciting the date or the name of the president. Doing
so early on in mild dementia may actually be a humane and compassionate practice, reorienting someone who can still retain information. This "reality therapy" is helpful early on. In 1990 I saw a very
compassionate reality therapist sit twenty deeply forgetful people on
chairs and stand up at a whiteboard to write the year in big blue letters. "What year is this," he asked. No one answered. "It's 1990!" he
exclaimed, and only one person responded with "Oh yes, 1990." No
harm was done, of course, and this gave people something to do. But
these days were we to gather deeply forgetful people together in that
room it would be instead to stimulate and engage them with a reading by an Alzheimer's poet, and most of them would chime in with a
smile to a deeply learned and meaningful verse after it was repeated
and sung a few times.

Caregivers for the deeply forgetful undeniably experience much
loss and anguish. And yet they demonstrate strength and resilience
because they have love. In his classic work, *Dementia Reconsidered:
The Person Comes First* (1997), my old friend Tom Kitwood defines

love within the context of dementia care as including comfort in the original sense of tenderness, closeness, the calming of anxiety, and bonding. Kitwood defines the primary psychological needs of persons with dementia in terms of care or love. He draws on the narratives of caregivers to assert that persons with dementia want love, "a generous, forgiving and unconditional acceptance, a wholehearted emotional giving, without any expectation of direct reward." The first component of that love is comfort, which includes tenderness, the calming of anxiety, and feelings of security based on affective closeness. Attachment, the second component of love, includes the formation of specific bonds that enhance a feeling of security. Inclusion in social experiences, and sharing activities that draw on a person's abilities, powers, and, finally, identity are other important components of love.

Each time we approach a deeply forgetful person with a kindly tone of voice and a reassuring facial expression, and call them by name with a smile, we are participating in an intervention that is as significant as any biotechnical one of which I am aware. It is the compassionate caregivers who remain the best hope for the deeply forgetful—and the rest of humankind—as they are role models for kindness in the world. Caregivers are the beacons of hope to be acknowledged and celebrated in their depth of commitment. They sway the social scale toward goodness not with single great acts of love but rather with daily small actions done in a spirit of great love. The dehumanization of medical care is apparent everywhere. Can we possess, and express, the unflinching self-awareness, empathic skills, and gratitude for the privilege of caring for the deeply forgetful that exemplify the healing art? The primary goals of every encounter with a person who is deeply forgetful should be these three things: to *accept, affirm, and connect.*

Accept   When Jim placed his twig in my hands, I accepted his gesture rather than reject it as meaningless.

Affirm   I smiled back at him and said that I was grateful as I held his twig.

Connect   I handed the twig back to him and listened to him utter the words "God is love." I then asked the nurse about the meaning of the twig.

Our dignity as human beings is at stake. We should question the increasing powers of biotechnology with regard to the modification and supposed "enhancement" of human nature itself, for biotechnology cannot by any means ensure the kind of self-improvement of heart that rests at the very center of human dignity. Developments like Botox, anabolic steroids, genetic modification (to make us faster and stronger), human growth hormone (to make our children a little taller—after daily injections over several years), and the promise of a fountain of youth do not qualify as contributors to our human dignity (Post and Binstock 2004). Rather, our dignity as human beings is ours to claim when we treat another person with love—expressed in celebration and attentive listening, creativity and helping, loyalty and respect. We can only preserve our own dignity as we conserve the dignity of the deeply forgetful.

The first principle of love for persons with cognitive disability is to reveal to them their value by providing attention, concern, and tenderness. Any experienced carer knows that the person with dementia, however advanced, will usually respond better to someone whose affect is affirming in tone.

It is the tone of our words, our facial expressions, and our actions that draw the cognitively disabled into the light of love. And through this exchange we discover that the disabled can still smile and appreciate our affirming presence.

Conclusions

For any caregiver who is running empty on hope, I suggest the following:

1. Have one Music and Memory session each day for about fifteen minutes to remind yourself that your loved one is "alive inside" and "still there" beneath the surface. Go to the Music & Memory website (www.musicandmemory.org) for details. Basically, play your loved one some music that they enjoyed years ago and identified with. Use an iPod. Watch your loved one get engaged with the rhythm. You will see this in body motion. They will begin to hum, and then chime in with a few lines or even whole verses. Afterward, for a few minutes, they may be able to respond to a simple question or two. This is good for them but great for you as a caregiver because you see that you are not caring for a shell.

2. Read favorite poetry that your loved one is familiar with and will likely respond to. Choose poems that meant something to them earlier in life. Try Robert Frost's "The Road Not Taken."

3. Call the local Alzheimer's Association and ask if they have a list of respite volunteers who can stop by for a few hours and give you a break for shopping, a walk in the park, or whatever you might need. Some faith communities provide this service. With a respite caregiver in the home for at least a half day once a week visit an art museum, catch up with an old trusted friend, and do something fun.

4. Definitely try a dementia support dog, as this is a huge positive for a lot of deeply forgetful people.

5. Do a daily stress-busting spiritual practice of relaxing mindfulness meditation or any form of focused mental attention

including reading. Get away from the pressures that create anxiety and stress.

6. Attend an Alzheimer's support group where you can process your feelings in a small group of a half-dozen other caregivers, with perhaps one facilitator. This should be a circle of trust, confidentiality, and empathic response where anyone feels free and safe to express anything.

7. With your loved one attend whatever creative arts programs for deeply forgetful people are available in the community. Notice what your loved one draws and ask them simple questions from time to time about any repeated images. This often brings a response.

8. Do not try to be a super-carer. Only try to manage difficult behaviors with the help of a good clinical social worker, an occupational therapist, or someone who knows how to work through these episodes.

9. Take care of your own health needs because caregiving is stressful and time-consuming, and it can wear you down.

10. Involve your faith community if you have one, including clinical pastoral care. It is also a good idea to sing familiar little tunes, like "You Are My Sunshine" or "Morning Has Broken." For folks with a religious history, sing old deeply learned hymns. And try to bring your loved one to a worship service because there is a strong possibility they will really get involved with the music and the prayers that they knew since childhood. Even small moments of connection can be very rewarding. Be always open to surprises. "Love never fails."

11. Use objects and art to connect to the underlying self. Use a book of interesting pictures of famous people like Marilyn Monroe or Joe DiMaggio, or landmarks like the Lincoln Memorial. Use objects to touch, or something nice to smell or taste (actually, a bit of chocolate works well).

Caregivers for individuals with Alzheimer's do in general have somewhat higher rates of depression than the general population, and some die before the individuals that they are caring for, presumably because they are stressed while the person with dementia is living mainly, but not entirely, in the pure present. Thus, hope is for the caregiver a crucial protective dynamic; their engagement with the continuing self-identity of a forgetful loved one may not bring full flourishing, but it can greatly increase their well-being.

Hopeful but realistic thinking is a part of the life of any caregiver, as it must be for any individual diagnosed with Alzheimer's while still in the early stages and capable of meaningful reflection. They know that there will be no big miracles. But they can find small miracles of self-expression if they are willing to look deep enough. And these small miracles are always also large ones in their power to infuse the spirit of the caregiver with immense meaning and hope.

Because I write for caregivers, many of whom have spiritual beliefs, rather than for scientists alone, I can afford to leave open a final question: Are we human beings who have spiritual experiences, or spiritual beings having a human experience? Caregivers may find hope in some perceived eternal soul in each of us, in which case maybe that loved one who seems so distant much of the time is still fully and firmly intact on some spiritual plane of consciousness about which we can have doubts, but not express them. In Buddhist cultures such as those of China and Japan, and in Hindu cultures as well, the deeply forgetful are thought to be on the path of detachment and enlightenment. Maybe that person, now very near the end, has already hopped on some mythical last train for glory, but it just hasn't quite left the station yet.

3

Answers to Sixteen Questions
Caregivers Ask from Diagnosis to Dying

I am fresh from a hospital in a local New York hamlet, where a ninety-year-old woman was crying out as if in agony all day. She is in the end stage of Alzheimer's. The hospital staff had put a plastic face piece over her mouth and nose, with a breathing tube of some kind down her throat. She was moaning when I arrived at 8 a.m., and all through the day patients in nearby rooms listened to her loud cries of pain. Her two adult children insisted that she be kept alive. We had a conversation about why they wanted her treated this aggressively. It turned out that they simply could not bear the idea of letting her pass away, because she was a fighter and she would have wanted to fight against death to the end. I listened quietly and with an empathic curiosity. Eventually I asked them about her apparent suffering and if there was any value in her being so tormented. They acknowledged that her moaning bothered them, but still their mom was a fighter, she loved life, and she had told them over the years before her dementia set in that they should do all they could to keep her alive. So they were adamant that she continue on with treatment that seemed to range between assault and torture. There was nothing I could do to persuade them to reconsider, sadly. After a little more conversation I left the room. Her daughter offered this as I was leaving: "She is only moaning because she has dementia, not because she is uncomfortable with her treatment."

Someday hopefully all such souls will be set free from the technologies that are sometimes still imposed on them, with a tube in their throat or belly and a butterfly needle in their veins. At every medical school where I have taught, students have regularly confided about how depressing it is for them to see the numbers of deeply forgetful people strapped into the intensive care unit beds, dying in a frightening metallic universe with buzzers and beepers sounding, and nothing to comfort them like the sounds of music in a hospice. Some students have lost sleep over such overtreatment and shared this with their peers in our reflection rounds. It is as though autonomous technology has taken these deeply forgetful people in its rough grip and held them gasping until their dying breath. What a dreadful way to pass on. But it happens because some family members refuse to let go, especially adult children who feel guilty if they do not have everything done that can be done.

Since 1990 I have worked with deeply forgetful people and their caregivers across all fifty states in the United States and all the provinces in Canada through community dialogues, focus groups, and ethics panels organized in collaboration with local Alzheimer's Association chapters (Post 1998) and coordinated through the national association's policy division in Washington, DC, thanks to Stephen McConnell and Michael Splaine. These panels and the writings that emanated from them led to the establishment of national ethics committees and guidelines in several countries including the United States and Canada (Cohen et al. 1999). As of 2021 I am continuing this work, most recently by contributing conferences on the one-fifth of deeply forgetful people who live alone or in relative isolation.

Over these three decades of responding to many inspirational caregivers like May (chapter one) and Orien Reid (chapter two), I have never thought that I had any knowledge myself that was not primarily formed by attentive listening to them with all their experience and real wisdom, and by a commitment to provide them with emotional support and kindness. I learned a great deal from caregivers about the ethical issues that arise with Alzheimer's from diagnosis to dying, and the sometimes hard facts of behavioral difficulties. In this chapter I will review the full range of issues that arise along the continuum of Alzheimer's disease, and in doing so will rely on the work of the Alzheimer's Association National Ethics Committee, upon which I once served.

Alzheimer's as a Cause of "Dementia"

Before proceeding with medical ethics, a point made earlier bears repetition: Alzheimer's is a disease that causes "dementia," but the syndrome (technically, a cluster of related symptoms) of dementia can have many other causes. A century ago the major cause of dementia was syphilis, a disease that progressed to the brain and/or heart in the absence of antibiotics, which became widely available in the early 1950s. Dementia can also be caused by trauma to the brain, as with chronic traumatic encephalitis (CTE), now familiar to many more people thanks to the movie *Concussion*. Actually, a concussion is not at all necessary for CTE to develop—constant head butts over the years will suffice. Many cases of Alzheimer's in males are mixed with CTE. There are other forms of dementia, as well. Vascular dementia—often called "multi-infarct dementia"—is caused by small stroke events, generally in the white matter of the brain, that go undetected in older adults until they accumulate and reach a certain level, although this form of dementia is generally more stable compared with Alzheimer's. In frontotemporal dementia, damage is focused in the front part of the brain, affecting personality and behavior more than memory, at least at first. Parkinson's disease too will generally involve dementia at some point. Alzheimer's is one of many causes of dementia, and it is also the most frequent cause nowadays—responsible for about 60 percent to 70 percent of all cases—because of our longer life expectancies, with age in and of itself as the main risk factor for Alzheimer's. So, *while all cases of Alzheimer's are a form of dementia, dementia itself is a much broader category, and a case of dementia may have nothing to do with Alzheimer's.*

Dementia as a general syndrome need not be progressive, meaning it need not worsen over time, but all cases of Alzheimer's involve some significant progression to a more advanced state, although we can never anticipate at what rate in any individual case, and we are never sure what capabilities will be affected or to what degree. Exceptions to this uncertainty are the two very rare (about 1 percent to 2 percent of all cases) early-onset familial forms of Alzheimer's, which usually progress rapidly from around age thirty-five or forty and lead to death within four or five years. With regard to the usual older-age Alzheimer's cases, by age sixty about 2 percent of older adults have probable Alzheimer's, and this percentage doubles every five years, so that by age seventy-five the incidence is close to 14 percent and continues to rise with each passing year. But it is hard to predict the rate of progression because Alzheimer's is often mixed with vascular dementia. As one senior neurologist who shied away from any generalizations about the progression of Alzheimer's told me, "Well, Stephen, you seen one case you seen one case." Each case is different, and so you never know (Devi 2017).

People with old-age Alzheimer's live an average of eight to ten years from diagnosis, *but almost nothing is more useless to the individual than averages*; some live up to twenty years or even more with highly varied quality of life, and some live only five or six years or even less. Changes in the brain at the cellular level may begin as many as twenty years or more before symptoms manifest. This constitutes a "preclinical phase," during which a variety of lifestyle modifications consistent with vascular health and a good diet might possibly delay onset, although this theory is as yet unproven (Devi 2017). Between the preclinical phase and actual onset of Alzheimer's there is supposedly a period of "mild cognitive impairment" before what is described as a "mild" stage; there is then a "moderate" stage that can last many years and will vary widely with regard to quality of life; and then an "advanced" or "terminal" stage that may last a couple of years or slightly more. But these stages have very little relevance for each unique individual. Changes in personality and behavior, and declines in memory, in the ability to speak and understand, to handle money, to recognize familiar faces, and various other losses are typical as the brain deteriorates, but these symptoms vary tremendously and manifest in every possible combination (Devi 2017).

With these definitions and distinctions stated, we can turn now to the ethical questions involved in caring for the deeply forgetful, of which there are many. I discuss sixteen of them in this chapter, but this list is not exhaustive. I have provided an answer to each question based on my experience working with the deeply forgetful as a starting point for reflection and based also on various discussions with graduate and medical students and professionals of all types.

Answers to Sixteen Questions

Based on our dialogues over decades and across four continents, these are the big questions, as caregivers have asked them.

Q1: Should we break the news to Grandma?

A1: Usually.

Diagnostic truth-telling in the context of dementia is ethically complex. In general, truth-telling should be handled as it is in other medical contexts: be as truthful as information permits while attending to the patient's need for social, emotional, spiritual, and practical support. A diagnosis of dementia is usually clear, but the precise cause can be "mixed"; for example, Alzheimer's and vascular dementia may appear together, perhaps with some chronic traumatic encephalitis involved due to repeated head injuries earlier in life. Even a diagnosis of Alzheimer's is always probable and usually accurate about 80 to 90 percent of the time. Alzheimer's is the cause of 60 to 70 percent of cases of dementia.

Compassionate diagnostic disclosure is considered a moral act of respect for persons in modern Western cultures, and indeed it is an opportunity to strengthen resilience and build community, as well as a necessary practical step in planning for the future. It takes compassionate care to break the news supportively, but it can be done with grace. My observation over the years is that individuals can be sensitively informed with clarity that they have dementia and manage that news, but "Alzheimer's" can be more difficult for them to handle, as the "A" word is so dreaded.

In the ethics panels I have served on across the United States and Canada, panels made up of leading physicians and other health professionals caring for those with dementia, as well as family caregivers and their deeply forgetful loved ones, almost everyone agrees that compassionate honesty is the best policy. There are disagreements about the optimal kinds of emotional and relational support, about precise timing of introducing the "A" word if it is to be used, and about whether to always inform the patient and their family together, or in some cases separately and sequentially.

Many experienced health care professionals have agonized about whether to tell a patient about Alzheimer's only to have the patient say, once they do, "That's what I've thought all along."

A good thing to say to a patient, and their family if they are present, might be something more or less like this:

> We know that you have some deep memory loss that is significant. It could remain at this level, but it may get more challenging for you with time. Let's wait and see. We have no crystal ball about these things and every case is unique. We will follow you closely, and on your next visit we can begin to talk about what could be causing this. It could be a lot of things. We may set you up for a couple of diagnostic tests just to learn more, okay? Do you have any questions?

As I indicated above, it is most often a good idea not to use the "A" word at this early stage of diagnosis, but as the diagnosis evolves it may be appropriate.

For many patients, hearing the "A" word is quite liberating because they are no longer confused about what is happening with them, and they can even let friends know that there is a reason why they may seem distant and forgetful. I knew a man in Cleveland named Murray who went door to door in his old neighborhood somewhat gleefully telling his neighbors that he was not being rude or detached—he had Alzheimer's (Post 2000).

Even if a diagnosis of probable Alzheimer's is eventually made, truth-telling is not an absolute. Certain cultures, especially many Asian American ones, do not embrace truth-telling as a norm when it comes to such a diagnosis, especially when they have larger doubts about the existence of Alzheimer's disease. They recognize that many older adults eventually can become senile, and they even expect it, but they view this more as a natural part of life and tend not to want to view it as a medical matter.

Some reasons for nondisclosure can be valid in certain cases.

The first is to protect a patient from anxiety, but this thinking underestimates the human capacity to deal creatively and resiliently with the implications of serious diagnoses and denies the power of a caring family or community to provide emotional healing. Many affected individuals, when provided with a diagnosis, are actually relieved of the anxiety that stems from uncertainty. The ways in which people cope with a diagnosis need to be carefully examined and analyzed, but if we were to argue that anxiety-related behaviors generally justify nondisclosure, then in the final analysis no patient would be told of a serious diagnosis, with disastrous results. Knowing the diagnosis and its emotional challenges for the patient mobilizes family and community to provide the care and acceptance without which the patient will only experience further isolation.

Yet still, there are people who simply do not want to hear the "A" word because they cannot handle it and state a preference not to be told, in which case it is better to speak of memory loss.

The second possible reason for nondisclosure is a cultural one. As mentioned above, the physician may encounter some patients from cultures where nondisclosure to the patient is still the model, and families still operate in a highly "protective" manner. The physician will clearly want to take this approach into consideration as a matter of cultural sensitivity, but individuals often want diagnostic information despite cultural pressures to the contrary, and physicians should not presume to withhold information unless the patient specifically requests this. While practicing with cultural sensitivity is indeed vital, a clinician's professional commitment is ultimately to individuals and their stated preferences, some of which will inevitably be countercultural. Moreover, cultures can have moral blind spots that are only gradually eliminated through interacting with other traditions, including the tradition of diagnostic truth-telling based on the principle of human dignity. But for some cultures, human dignity requires protection from diagnostic truth-telling. It must be said too that a person who has Alzheimer's will get to a point where they have no insight into the meaning of the "A" word.

It never hurts to ask the patient, "Is this something you want me to tell you details about, or can we just say that your memory is fading and leave the rest up to your family?" Indeed, around the United States there are now many "memory disorder centers" that were once "Alzheimer's centers," in part to avoid overusing the dreaded "A" word. Memory loss is easier to speak of for many families and patients. Telling a person the truth about a diagnosis of progressive dementia caused by probable Alzheimer's or some other dementia-causing disease is generally consistent with the principle of respect for persons in Western cultures and should be valued as such. But it is *not* the responsibility of clinicians to transform cultures so much as to understand and honor them. The modern fields of clinical bioethics and medical law emphasize truth-telling and informed consent, and rightly so, but such truth-telling can be in clear tension with important cultural sensitivities that need to be respected.

Truth-telling is important as a right that allows patients and their families to plan for the future, financially and otherwise. This seems absolutely necessary for the "live alones," people with dementia who have no families and live on their own. Informing individuals about their diagnosis allows them to decide how most to enjoy the remaining years of relatively unimpaired mental functioning. An important Alzheimer's Association statement (2001) includes the argument that disclosing the diagnosis early in the illness process allows the person to "be involved in communicating and planning for end-of-life decisions." Certainly diagnostic truth-telling is the precondition for the ethics of "precedent autonomy" for those who wish to gain control over their futures through advance directives. Such directives include durable power of attorney for health care, which allows a trusted loved one to make any and all treatment decisions once the agent becomes incompetent, and it can effectively be coupled with a living will or some other specific indication of the agent's wishes with regard to end-of-life care. Unless the affected person knows their probable diagnosis while still competent to file such legal instruments, the risk that they will be subjected to burdensome medical technologies is increased.

Perhaps most important, disclosure permits the person with dementia to participate in counseling and support group interventions, thus helping to alleviate anger, self-blame, fear, and depression (Riley 1989).

The diagnosis of dementia does have stigma associated with it in the popular culture, and stigma is the beginning point of de-dignifying. When a major public figure "comes out" with a diagnosis of Alzheimer's and speaks honestly of their hopes, the stigma may be at least somewhat alleviated. This is why President Ronald Reagan announced his diagnosis of Alzheimer's openly to the American people in a letter that appeared November 11, 1994, on the front page of virtually every newspaper in the nation and around the world. By using the word Alzheimer's publicly, President Reagan contributed to a changing of attitudes. He helped lift the veil of secrecy and shame associated with this disease and, in so doing, helped liberate many diagnosed persons and their families from a prison of silence and stigma. President Reagan wrote as follows:

My fellow Americans:

I have recently been told that I am one of the millions of Americans who will be afflicted with Alzheimer's disease.

Upon learning this news, Nancy and I had to decide whether as private citizens we would keep this a private matter or whether we would make this news known in a public way.

In the past Nancy suffered from breast cancer and I had my cancer surgeries. We found that through our open disclosures we were able to raise public awareness. We were happy that as a result many more people underwent testing. They were treated in early stages and able to return to normal, healthy lives. So now we feel it is important to share it with you. In opening our hearts, we hope this might promote greater awareness of this condition. Perhaps it will encourage a clearer understanding of the individuals and families who are affected by it.

At the moment I feel just fine. I intend to live the remainder of the years God gives me on this earth doing the things I have always done. I will continue to share life's journey with my beloved Nancy and my family. I plan to enjoy the great outdoors and stay in touch with my friends and supporters.

Unfortunately, as Alzheimer's disease progresses, the family often bears a heavy burden. I only wish there was some way I could spare Nancy from this painful experience. When the time comes I am confident that with your help she will face it with faith and courage.

In closing let me thank you, the American people, for giving me the great honor of allowing me to serve as your president. When the Lord calls me home, whenever that may be, I will leave with the greatest love for this country of ours and eternal optimism about its future.

I now begin the journey that will lead me into the sunset of my life. I know that for America there will always be a bright dawn ahead.

Thank you, my friends. May God always bless you.

Sincerely,
Ronald Reagan

When physicians inform affected individuals and their families about the diagnosis of probable Alzheimer's—as they usually should do on the second or third visit if they have a fairly clear diagnosis—the communication of the diagnosis should usually occur in a joint meeting with the affected individual and their family to provide the individual with emotional support. Almost without exception, affected individuals and their family members approach clinicians together, in order to jointly understand the diagnosis and its implications for the future of the family unit. Hence, except in cases when the individual objects to sharing his or her diagnosis with the family, confidentiality is seldom a concern. Even when a patient has only limited support, however, disclosure is appropriate. Most individuals already sense that their routine functioning is diminished and are frustrated by poor recall and/or a reduced ability to express themselves.

It is also important that the content, timing, and manner of disclosure are appropriate for the affected person and family, consistent with variations in culture and cultural values as well as with the physician's knowledge of the specific family dynamics. Disclosure of the diagnosis should allow sufficient time for questions from family members and from the person diagnosed, as well as for recommendations from the physician and health care team. It is helpful to include in the family meeting an additional member of the team, such as a social worker or nurse, who can answer questions and discuss recommendations and resources. A follow-up session is beneficial to further discuss the diagnosis and available support systems.

As a result of this communication process, the affected person and their family should come to understand:

> This degree of memory loss is not normal but results
>   from changes in the brain.
> Expectations for the future are uncertain, but in general,
>   there will be further loss of memory.

> While the disease cannot be cured, many of its effects
>   can be treated.
>
> Having Alzheimer's does not mean that you cannot enjoy
>   many experiences and retain your selfhood.
>
> Support groups, such as those sponsored by the Alzheimer's
>   Association, are available and effective.
>
> The health care team will be available to provide assistance
>   throughout the disease process, although your quality of life
>   will really depend almost entirely on nonmedical factors.
>   (Foley and Post 1993)

With diagnostic disclosure comes the responsibility to direct the affected individual and family to available resources. A specific care plan should be discussed and agreed upon. Nurses and social workers can be especially helpful during such discussions. Emphasis should be placed on the health care team's availability to give direct assistance or to make referrals. Although the patient's dementia cannot be cured, the team should emphasize the fact that efforts will be made to treat its effects and to assist the affected person and family in coping with the illness.

Q2: How quickly will I decline?

A2: This varies greatly from person to person, and some cases are much better than others, but there will be further decline.

As I have already pointed out, when it comes to Alzheimer's, every case is different. The rate of progression and the capacities affected vary; depending on the individual progression, some capacities will be largely spared, while others will not. Genetics, vascular health, diet, brain reserve, areas of the brain affected, stress, quality of psychosocial interactions, and other factors all play a part in determining the nature and rate of progression. Some brains are more resilient than others because they have more connective "synapses," or gaps, between the tips of cells across which communicative chemicals (neurotransmitters) pass. A probable diagnosis of Alzheimer's allows the physician to state on a second or third visit, "You have a form of dementia that seems likely to be of the progressive Alzheimer's type, but we really do not know how quickly or how much it will progress, and it can be surprisingly stable for years."

A thoughtful neurologist who cares compassionately for deeply forgetful people, Dr. Gayatri Devi, likens Alzheimer's to the autism "spectrum" in that there are many forms and they are all a little different, so you never quite know how any individual will be affected (Devi 2017). And of course, a person with Alzheimer's can be doing reasonably well, but then a sudden shift of environment—such as admission to a hospital for a hip fracture surgery—might cause a precipitous decline. (In general, surgery for patients with dementia can and should be avoided.)

When it comes to Alzheimer's, *no one can predict exactly how or how rapidly an individual will be affected* other than in the most generic terms, such as "this will worsen, but you can still have valuable and meaningful years ahead." The most important reason to avoid stereotypes and overly concrete stage theories of the disease generally, however, is that they divert attention from *the moral challenge of Alzheimer's, which is to focus on the uniqueness of each individual, and to remain undaunted in providing the psychosocial-environmental opportunities that are clearly the best current treatment available for these patients.* We need to bear in mind that even for those growing old and a bit senile, small gratifications can be very important, and life can still be worth living (Devi 2017).

One way touted by some people to prevent onset of Alzheimer's or to slow a person's decline is a combination of the Mediterranean diet, greens and fruits, regular exercise, social and intellectual engagement, peaceful walks with friends, and playing games like checkers or doing a crossword puzzle. Meditation against stress is also helpful (see www.alzheimersprevention.org).

Q3: Are there really any effective drugs to stop this disease?

A3: Not so much, but you can try out what is available.*

On a scale of 1 to 10, if insulin rates a 9 as an effective drug to treat diabetes, what we have to date for Alzheimer's is very roughly a 1. Alzheimer's is extremely complex, and researchers trying to develop an effective treatment have found it one of the toughest diseases to decipher. Even after decades of investigation success is nowhere in sight, although there is greater hope now that more talented researchers are focused on it than ever before.

There are about one hundred billion neurons (brain cells) in an average adult brain, with branches that connect at more than one hundred trillion points, like trees intermingling in a huge "neuron forest." Signals—electrical charges—traveling through the neuron forest form the basis of memories, thoughts, and feelings. Neurons connect to one another at synapses, or infinitesimally small gaps, and when a signal reaches a synapse it may trigger the release of tiny bursts of chemicals called neurotransmitters that travel across the synapse carrying signals to other cells.

Alzheimer's disrupts both the way the electrical charges travel within cells and the activity of neurotransmitters at these gaps, even-

---

* Response provided with the assistance of Gregg Cantor, MD, Stony Brook University Medical Center.

tually leading to cell death and tissue loss. Scientists have continued to debate what actually causes this disruption. Some think it may be due to "plaques" that build up between neurons, and/or "tangles" that build up within them. Plaques are "sticky" clumps of protein (molecules composed of forty-two amino acids) that form tangles inside the cells and block cell-to-cell signaling at the synapses; they also trigger an immune response that results in inflammation. In healthy cells, tau protein provides a supportive strand-like matrix for the tracks within the cell over which food molecules, cell parts, and other key materials are thought to travel. In cells where plaque develops those tracks disintegrate into tangles, so supplies can no longer travel over them to nourish and repair the individual cell, and the plaques and tangles tend to spread through the cortex as the disease progresses. Another complicating factor is that many people with lots of plaques and tangles visible at autopsy showed no symptoms of Alzheimer's at all before they died, so many good researchers now doubt that either plaques or tangles cause Alzheimer's and see them instead as downstream aftereffects.

Some doctors may or may not write a lot of prescriptions for the available Alzheimer's medications, but those who do are responding to the American tendency to place hope in magic bullets. Other doctors think that existing drug treatments are a pointless waste of resources. It is reasonable to give drugs a try, but it is also reasonable to avoid them or to stop taking them at some point, because they do have side effects and cost money while providing few if any demonstrable benefits—other than to the bottom line of the pharmaceutical corporations that produce them.

Acetylcholinesterase Inhibitors

In order to treat Alzheimer's, whether early- or late-onset, researchers have focused on manipulating the levels of specific neurotransmitters in the synapses, but this approach has not worked out terribly well, despite some initial excitement. Increases in acetylcholine were thought to improve memory function, and tacrine, which in 1993 became the first drug approved by the FDA for treating mild and moderate Alzheimer's disease, limited the natural breakdown of the neurotransmitter acetylcholine in the synapses. A large trial in 1994 found that increasing the levels of acetylcholine from tacrine use led to "a significant and clinically observed improvement on objective cognitive tests, clinician- and caregiver-rated global evaluations, and quality-of-life assessments" (Knapp, Knopman, and Solomon 1994, 989). However, such claims have more recently been viewed as exaggerations. Though this study showed that some people had small improvements in word-finding and attention in the early phase of Alzheimer's, even these benefits were hardly if at all significant, disappeared quickly, and had absolutely no impact on the underlying progression of the disease. Moreover, many people in this study had to stop taking the drug due to harmful side effects, such as a rise in liver enzymes (Knapp, Knopman, and Solomon 1994). As a result, tacrine was discontinued.

Some years later, more acetylcholinesterase inhibitors became available. But still, prescribing these drugs is a bit like treating a brain tumor with aspirin. Of course, neurologists do sometimes prescribe aspirin for patients with a brain tumor to help alleviate symptoms, but this obviously has no impact on the underlying tumor itself. For example, in 1996 a new acetylcholinesterase inhibitor called donepezil was approved. Following the approval of donepezil, two other drugs in the same class of medications became available—rivastigmine (in 2000), and galantamine (in 2001). The three new drugs had no toxic side effects, but donepezil for one can cause diarrhea, vomiting, nausea, dizziness, drowsiness, weakness, trouble sleeping, and shakiness (tremor) while adjusting to the drug, and gastrointestinal discomfort can be significant enough that as many as one in five people have to discontinue use. These drugs remain relatively ineffective. Of the three, donepezil is currently approved for all stages of Alzheimer's disease (mild, moderate, and severe), while galantamine and rivastigmine are approved only for the mild and moderate stages. Donepezil was originally approved only for the early stage, but aggressive marketing in nursing homes along with the dubious assertion that going off the drug would cause a dramatic decline or behavioral problems resulted in its being overused. An analysis of thirteen randomized industry-funded trials that compared these drugs to a placebo initially showed very modest improvements, all of which are questionable. These improvements were measured by assessing patients at six to twelve months using a number of different scales: a seventy-point Alzheimer's Assessment Scale-Cognitive Subscale, the Mini-Mental State Examination (MMSE), the patients' functioning in activities of daily living (ADLs), and global impression of the patients by their caretakers (Courtney 2004). The results of these assessments showed that the benefits of donepezil, rivastigmine, and galantamine for activities of daily living are rather unsubstantial, and their cognitive benefits are even less obvious. Because these drugs appear to offer little benefit to patients who take them, it is also a myth that patients who stop taking them suffer some precipitous decline.

Furthermore, even though this meta-analysis demonstrated some very slight benefits with these drugs, other studies show no benefits at all. For instance, the AD2000 study, which was different from the above-mentioned studies in that it was not industry funded, showed no significant difference between using a placebo versus an acetylcholinesterase inhibitor in terms of entry to institutional care, progression of disability, or psychological symptoms (Courtney 2004). Because it was independently conducted, the AD2000 study stirred debate about the effectiveness of acetylcholinesterase inhibitors for the treatment of Alzheimer's, and some European countries stopped providing them through their national health services. Unfortunately, despite the fact that this class of drugs is still the backbone of Alzheimer's disease treatment in most places, the results in patients using them continue to be insignificant. And because of such limited outcomes, the pharmaceutical companies, having made their billions, have now started exploring other biological pathways.

NMDA Receptor Antagonists

A newer drug, approved by the FDA in 2003 for the treatment of moderate to severe Alzheimer's, is memantine. Instead of targeting acetylcholine, memantine targets and antagonizes the N-methyl-D-aspartate (NMDA) receptor for the neurotransmitter glutamate. Just as with the studies of acetylcholinesterase inhibitors, however, the major studies of memantine resulted in controversial findings regarding its effects. One trial split 295 patients with moderate to severe Alzheimer's into four groups (no-therapy group, donepezil-only group, memantine-only group, and donepezil-and-memantine group) to see which group would show the greatest benefit (Howard et al. 2012). After one year, the patients taking memantine scored higher on the Mini-Mental State Exam (MMSE); however, they scored lower on the Bristol Activities of Daily Living Scale. Overall, the average differences in scores among the four groups were considered to be not clinically significant (Howard et al. 2012).

Ask About the Side Effects and
Know You Can Stop Medications Anytime

The most common side effects of the acetylcholinesterase inhibitors include insomnia, nausea, diarrhea, dizziness, falls, and infection in more than 10 percent of those who take them. Memantine, on the other hand, has been shown to cause dizziness, confusion, hallucinations, diarrhea, infection, and urinary incontinence in 1 percent to 10 percent of patients.

These medications can also impose a heavy financial burden on patients. Memantine can cost an average of $450 to $500 for a one-month supply, while generic acetylcholinesterase inhibitors cost on average $200 to $250 per month.

While an effective drug to slow or halt the progression of Alzheimer's continues to be sought, there are drugs available in the meantime to help with agitation, combativeness, hallucinations, and aggression should these behaviors arise in some patients during the moderate stage of the disease, although such problems often can, and ideally will, be managed by improvements in the patient's environmental, communicative, and social situation.

Some affected individuals may experience, and express, a burst of renewed self-confidence in their cognitive capacities after taking any new compound, whether artificial or natural. But how much of this perceived improvement is due to the compound itself remains unclear. Presumably each person with Alzheimer's is a part of some relational network that inevitably plays a role in the patient's self-perception; indeed, self-perception is highly dependent on the perceptions of others, especially caregivers, who are always in need of even a small glimmer of hope.

It is hard for doctors to know how to respond to patients' and caregivers' passion for the possible. Should unrealistic hopes be indulged for emotional reasons? Should the money expended for new compounds of relatively marginal efficacy be spent instead on improving the patient's environment and expanding his or her relational opportunities? Medication needs to be situated within a full program of dementia care (including emotional, relational, and environmental interventions) so that it is not relied on excessively; family members should be respected when they want to stop a patient's medication; and even when medication is desired, families need to appreciate the limits of current compounds.

To sum up, decisions about the medications currently available to treat Alzheimer's are ethically and financially complex because their efficacy is quite limited, the affected individual remains on the inevitable downward trajectory of irreversible progressive dementia, and there may be nonchemical interventions focused on emotional, relational, and spiritual well-being that are both cheaper and more effective. This is not to suggest that we should all be pharmacological Calvinists rather than pharmacological hedonists, but pharmaceutical companies wield too great an influence on various Alzheimer's organizations.

Given that there is no known impact in presymptomatic use of cholinesterase drugs in people with mild cognitive impairment (pre-Alzheimer's memory loss converting to dementia in a few years), and that these drugs do little to slow and absolutely nothing to reverse Alzheimer's even in combination with a glucose antagonist, what are they good for? They may delay nursing home placement a bit, but what happens once the patient is in the nursing home? There is no convincing evidence that taking people off drugs speeds decline. So perhaps we would benefit deeply forgetful people more by providing them with supporting music and dogs.

Multiple biologies, multiple genetics, multiple ages of onset, multiple rates of progressions—this suggests a spectrum disorder and possibly even different disease causes, so that Alzheimer's is a label being used too widely. As the basic science of Alzheimer's has progressed, scientists have had a hard time picking out the right targets of attack for new compounds.

In 2010, a National Institutes of Health panel, after reviewing the world's scientific literature, found that "currently, no evidence of even moderate scientific quality exists to support the association of any modifiable factor (such as nutritional supplements, herbal preparations, dietary factors, prescription or nonprescription drugs, social or economic factors, medical conditions, toxins, or environmental exposures) with reduced risk of Alzheimer's disease"—and this finding is still accurate today.

Q4: Can tender loving care make a difference,
      or is it all just biological?

A4: Yes indeed, because kindness can make
      things a lot less stressful.

In approaching Alzheimer's, any strict biological determinism is misguided; because the brain is always interacting with social and environmental factors, love and support can reduce stress and make a real difference in the patient's condition and disease progression (Devi 2017). Scientists describe neuroplasticity as the ability of the brain to produce new neurons and connections between them based on external circumstances and stimuli. Neurologist Gayatri Devi describes Alzheimer's as a spectrum disorder, with a wide range from very severe to much less severe. And she argues that kindness and a positive social outlook and engagement matter a lot.

Just as adverse psychosocial circumstances and related emotions and stress negatively affect the brain, so too can affirmation, kindness, social engagement, creativity, spiritual practice, and a pleasant environment positively affect the brain through neuroplasticity, and thus to some extent influence symptoms. So when we treat a deeply forgetful individual with respect and warmth, we are to some degree having an effect on their brain and encouraging the manifestation of lost capacities. Through our interactions with them we are either amplifying the individual's anxiety level or amplifying their sense of well-being. But in every sense, how we interact makes a difference, a fact supported by a study from the 1990s that first used the term "rementia" to describe a fleeting period of slight symptom improvement based on positive stimulations such as personalized music, poetry reading, artistic creativity, social engagement, and many other factors (Smith and Copeland 1993). Hence the immense popularity of Dan Cohen's Music and Memory programs for Alzheimer's patients, which reveal their remaining selfhood and capacity underneath the chaos through playing personalized music with which they identified closely earlier in life, or readings of poetry or other works that older adults will likely know, like Robert Frost's "The Road Not Taken." All of these activities demonstrate that while Alzheimer's disease is progressive, any individual can experience improvements in the context of eventual decline.

I want to emphasize again that there is a serious disadvantage in thinking of Alzheimer's in narrowly neurological terms, because doing so focuses us on biology alone rather than on the biopsychosocial dimensions of the illness experience, which can always be enhanced. The biomedical model has taken a pathological approach to Alzheimer's and focuses on the development of medications that to date have had no impressive effects, though that may change as we learn more about the disease. By focusing on the "war against Alzheimer's disease," this medicalization of Alzheimer's has also proved harmful because it has deflected our attention from all the nonmedical things that can and should be done and obscured all the ways in which we can bring benefit to the lives of deeply forgetful people. On too many occasions neurologists simply run a brain scan on a person struggling with memory loss, show the pictures of the brain on a screen, and tell the patient and family members that based on the images and other tests this is likely Alzheimer's, after which the typical routine focuses on prescribing what is at least to date some relatively inconsequential pill. Clearly, one important key to fulfilling the moral challenge of Alzheimer's is overcoming the adverse impact of a strictly biomedical model.

The bottom line: negative interactions have a negative effect on the brain, so the preferred prescription is a combination of dignity, respect, and kindness!

Q5: Should we tell other people about my diagnosis?

A6: Only tell people you trust.

When deciding whether to share a diagnosis of Alzheimer's, and with whom, it is important to keep in mind that one may experience discrimination or stigma as a result. Sabat has referred to this effect as "excess disability"—what happens when negative social attitudes and interactions cause a person's functional incapacity to exceed the level warranted by his or her actual impairment (Sabat 2000).

Creativity, mirth, relationship, dance, music, and joy are all possible for deeply forgetful people as those around them shift from correcting to connecting. But with whom you share a diagnosis depends entirely on your comfort level, and you need only confide in people that you know care for you and that you can trust.

Some people feel it is liberating to tell all their friends and neighbors about a diagnosis of probable Alzheimer's because it explains why they forget names, are perhaps emotionally disengaged and distant, or otherwise behave a little differently than they once did. Thus the man mentioned earlier in the chapter who went door to door happily announcing to his many close neighbors, "I know I have ignored you a few times when I passed you on the sidewalk, but guess what? I'm not a schmuck at all, it's just that I have a disease called Alzheimer's!"

Unfortunately, deeply forgetful people are vulnerable to malignant social psychology because of "hypercognitive values" (Post 1995b, 3), the tendency in Western culture to prioritize intellect and reason over all other aspects of meaningful human consciousness. I was initially moved to write this critique of hypercognitive values and Western liberal cultures because they inevitably cast deeply forgetful people in an overly negative light, describing the experience of dementia in exclusively negative terms. John Swinton summarized my work thus: "The tension between the hypercognitive cultural story with its expectations and demands for loss and devastation to be the prevailing script and a counter-story of love and possibilities couldn't be starker" (Swinton 2012, 82). In a hypercognitive culture, instead of building personhood we destroy it through neglect, disempowerment, intimidation, objectification, mockery, invalidation, and the like (Swinton 2012, 82).

Q6: Will "I" still be there, more or less, despite the silence or confusion?

A6: We can never say no, and caregivers notice the expressions of self-identity.

It is my observation that the best caregivers strive to both remind loved ones of their selfhood and to notice the expressions of such selfhood, however sporadic. They remain open to surprises, and they find meaning and hope in such moments. We must provide deeply forgetful people with cues, bringing them back to their selfhood using familiar music, images, poems, and art. Every caregiver can practice the art of revival, refreshing memories. Even the words of the caregiver are cues, chosen to suggest to a loved one the very words and names that they seem to have entirely forgotten. And then these caregivers celebrate these moments of revival with appreciation and affirmation.

Underneath the chaos, and evoked by reminders from others, by music, by social connections and interactions, there is always an "I" there—a continuity of selfhood and personal narrative—that reveals itself sporadically. But even when that narrative of selfhood is not being actively expressed, there is still a basic sense of "I" that can manifest in emotional reactions such as anger or rage in response to annoying interactions and discomforts. There can also be a wonderfully peaceful and quiet presence that conveys tranquility in the depths of forgetfulness.

The idea that there is "no self" is morally dangerous, because it implies that the deeply forgetful person has no moral status under the protective umbrella of the imperative to "do no harm." Instead, they are "already gone." In fact, empirical studies indicate that *all* participants with moderate dementia demonstrate self-recognition, and only 25 percent of study participants with moderately severe dementia did not recognize themselves (Fazio 2008, 58), so there is a sense of self and as such deeply forgetful people are to be respected like anyone else when it comes to daily preferences and choices as expressed explicitly or more subtly. Fazio's studies using mirrors show that self-recognition is the norm until Alzheimer's reaches a very advanced stage. Furthermore, Georgetown psychologist Steven R. Sabat has devoted years to carefully observing and interacting with people with advanced Alzheimer's, and through the methods of phenomenology demonstrates that the basic core sense of personal self-identity persists throughout the disease (Sabat 2018), as indicated among other things by participants' use of personal pronouns.

Thus, when we ask if an "I" is still there, the answer is very probably yes. Fazio concludes that based on both visual self-recognition and linguistic self-reference, aspects of the self that appear gone may be elicited by creating "environments and interactions that are reflective and supportive of a lifelong self, thus allowing it to persist in Alzheimer's care" (Fazio 2008, 70). Our task as caregivers then is to create a symbolic environment and a community around these individuals to remind them of who they are.

Rationality as a decisional capacity is not morally important in deeply forgetful people after a certain level of decline. It is rationality as a source of self-identity that matters—that is, "who" we are rather than "how" we proceed. And in this sense, the deeply forgetful can be surprising in response to the symbols around them.

Sabat notes that while physicians treating dementia attribute errors in speech and understanding to brain damage alone, he tends to view the problem as one of misunderstood communications, and he outlines the ways in which efforts at communication by those affected are more meaningful than we might assume at first glance. He also suggests techniques to improve communication, such as not interrupting, allowing for pauses, and word queuing. He describes the cognitive and social abilities of deeply forgetful people, their subjective experiences and intentionality, and discusses how behaviors otherwise considered meaningless reveal their intentions, interpretive capacity, and ability to evaluate different situations.

It would be difficult to exaggerate the significance of experiences of terminal lucidity, when an individual who has not spoken in months is nearing the end of life and on that final day surprises an old friend with a wonderful spoken treat. Dr. Joe Foley once visited an old friend he had known years earlier at the College of the Holy Cross. The friend, a priest, had eventually developed dementia and had spent a number of years in a nursing home; he was now in the end stages of Alzheimer's. Joe, who always treated people in this condition as he would anyone else, had been sitting with his old friend for several hours talking about how many wonderful experiences they had had together. Joe never expected responses, but he was always open to the possibility. Then, all of a sudden, his friend said, "Yes Joe, we had the most wonderful times together." And then he died.

Joe would always tell me this story to inspire hope, patience, and respect.

Q7:   Will I "suffer"?

A7:   No, because you will forget that you forget, and any physical pain can and should be alleviated.*

There is always suffering in the decline to old age, and a slow weaning from the things of the world that is accompanied by various degrees of anxiety and fear. But there can be freedom and a lightness of being as well. Think of Alzheimer's as aging into the moment, into the world of the pure present, free from the chronological glue that connects past and future. Sometimes, given the pressures of modern life, I feel free just being around deeply forgetful people because they bring me into the *now*—there is no other place to be with them. And when I meditate on them and their way of being, I sense that they perhaps already have one foot on the train to another world.

"Will I suffer?" Most of us are so horrified at the very idea of becoming deeply forgetful that we assume it entails a lot of suffering. But once a person gets to the point where they forget that they forget, anxiety and fear diminish, and they drift into the now. We

---

* Response provided with the assistance of Kathleen Culver, RN, Stony Brook University Medical Center Palliative Care.

assume that forgetfulness causes suffering because we are viewing this condition through the lens of hypercognitive values, or we sense that we somehow must remain more independent from others than we ever really were or can actually be, or we believe that we have to be earning a buck until our last day on earth to be fully human.

This is the result when, regrettably, we view dementia through a model of reality that requires a person to conform to particular rules of communication and social interaction. We suffer only when we continue to believe that we must adhere to the ways of the dominant culture, to be as we are "supposed" to be and behave as we are "supposed" to behave. It is for this reason that I have argued for years that the turning point in progressive dementia really comes when we "forget that we forget," and then peace is possible. Go with the flow.

As for physical pain, deeply forgetful people are as likely to suffer from it as any older adult (Hadjistavropoulos, Fitzgerald, and Marchildon 2010). Self-reporting of pain is considered the gold standard in pain assessment (Hadjistavropoulos et al. 2014), but self-reporting has limitations and is often impossible in advanced dementia, because of impaired cognitive, linguistic, and social skills. So observational pain assessment scales have been developed to evaluate elderly persons with cognitive issues. When using the Pain Assessment in Advanced Dementia (PAINAD) tool, an observer assigns a score of 0 to 2 across each of five domains to rate the patient's pain intensity on a total scale of 0 to 10. A skilled assessor can complete the scoring in less than two minutes (Kooten et al. 2017).

Note that in nursing homes about half of the residents generally have a form of dementia, and about half of them experience pain not from dementia itself, but from chronic arthritis, back issues, and other conditions. To assess pain, focus on PAINAD:

- breathing (labored, noisy, hyperventilating)

- vocalization (moaning, crying out)
- facial expression (frightened, frowning, grimacing)
- body language (curled up, clenched fists, tenseness, pushing away caregivers, rubbing)
- behaviors (agitation, irritability, screaming, sleeping patterns, loss of appetite, crying, wandering)

Q8: **Do I really want to continue to treat my heart failure or diabetes or dialysis or cancer as this disease unfolds?**

A8: **As a general suggestion, no.**

In general, those with dementia are as free as anyone else to stop whatever treatments they wish, so long as they have the capacity to make informed decisions. Then, by creating a living will, they can ensure that they will not be continuously treated should they not desire such treatment prospectively. Ongoing treatment can also be avoided by signing a durable power of attorney, or by the authority of family surrogate decision makers.

The key factor in determining when to end treatment is the minimization of physical suffering, and to a deeply forgetful person, something as simple as the insertion of a butterfly needle can be experienced as assault or torture. I recommend a very restrained approach when treating the other sorts of conditions listed above. In general, surgeries should not be performed. Palliative surgery might be advisable in some rare instances, but be aware that anesthesia will likely lead to accelerated cognitive decline. Sometimes treatment to shrink a tumor can be palliative, which makes sense. But in general, let cancer take its course. There is also usually no need for hip surgery that necessitates removal to a hospital, and CPR or intubation of any sort should be against the law. These are all just torturous to the vulnerable forgetful. A good natural dying may involve some assisted oral feeding, but avoid feeding tubes like the plague.

Likewise, there is no absolute imperative to treat a chest infection with antibiotics, especially one that has already recurred a few times, and in any case antibiotics will eventually become ineffective. But urinary tract infections should be treated with antibiotics to whatever extent possible for pain control. To sum up: when caring for the deeply forgetful, especially those with terminal conditions, there is no real need for any treatment that is other than palliative.

Q9: Will I be a burden to those
     who take care of me?

A9: Finding meaning and providing
    self-care are the keys for caregivers.[*]

Caregivers spend much of their time and energy tending to their loved one's needs, day and night—and often for years at a stretch. The psychosocial, physical, and financial effects of caregiving can be stressful and anxiety provoking, which negatively affects the quality of life for this group (Farina et al. 2017). Their feelings of hopelessness, loss, and isolation are well founded and should be acknowledged as a consequence of the very act of providing care to a loved one, often without receiving the traditional expressions of appreciation. But they can fail to see the importance of taking care of themselves, so it is necessary to convey to them the value in taking some time to do so. Finding respite care, accessing community support, knowing when to lean on others, and stepping aside at the right time to rely instead on professional help are all important aspects of care-

---

[*] Response provided with the assistance of Jennifer Kolar, RN, Stony Brook Medical Center.

giver self-care and self-maintenance. The positive effects of being able to recharge are notable after only a couple of days away, or even a couple of hours (Post 2007).

We also need to keep in mind that it takes a village to care for someone who is deeply forgetful, and the involvement of community is essential. Communities of faith should prioritize this as a mission area, as should many other organizations. The Alzheimer's Association support groups are already well established and provide a worthwhile service.

The implementation of caregiver training programs has also proven effective in decreasing burnout and depression. Many of these successful programs, such as Resources to Enhance Alzheimer's Caregiver Health VA, include education in disease progression, skills training, and psychoeducation (Cheng et al. 2016). By helping to reduce the frustrations inherent in caregiving, and by setting realistic goals for those involved in it, programs like these have also enabled participants to identify and experience some of the positive aspects of this work.

These results reflect broader increased interest in benefit-finding and in the importance of meaning-making for caregivers, with the ensuing positive effects on quality of life as they learn to savor moments of joy, communication, creativity, gratitude, and the like. The expanding field of positive psychology has encouraged a focus on understanding the lived experience as well as using it to find meaning and value in times of illness or during the golden years of one's life, in addition to enhancing the experience of caregivers. Applying positive psychosocial interventions has been shown to improve the well-being of dementia patients (Clarke and Wolverson 2016).

"The adaptation process of caregiving is characterized by the coexistence of both positive and negative experiences" (Yu, Cheng, and Wang 2018, 2). But while the negatives of caregiving get a lot of attention, the positives exist too and can manifest as moments of inspiration or renewed purpose, self-discovery, personal growth, and a feeling of connection with the person afflicted with Alzheimer's (Cheng et al. 2017). Such positive experiences are effective in lessening the burden of caregiving and the depression that often accompanies it.

Q10: Is genetic testing a good idea?

A10: Generally, it is not.

Genetic testing was frowned on in the statement issued in 2017 by the Alzheimer's Association (https://www.alz.org/media/Documents/genetic-testing-statement.pdf), except in early-onset familial cases where a single gene mutation causes the disease. There is really no clinical value in genetic testing once you are diagnosed with Alzheimer's disease; before diagnosis such testing would be useful only if the tests were clearly predictive and if there was something you could do with the information to prevent onset, like changing your lifestyle or accessing preventive medicine. At this time, however, no such medicine is available.

Alzheimer's is the subject of intense genetic analysis. It is a genetically heterogeneous disorder—meaning that, to date, it is associated with three determinative or causal gene mutations (someone who has that mutation will definitely get the disease) and one susceptibility or risk gene. The three causal Alzheimer's gene mutations (located on chromosomes 21, 14, and 1) were discovered in the late 1990s. These are autosomal-dominant genes and pertain to early-onset familial forms of Alzheimer's (usually manifesting between the late thirties and early forties) which, according to one estimate, account for less than 3 percent of all cases. These families are usually well aware of their unique histories. Only in these relatively few unfortunate families is genetic prediction actually possible, for those who carry the mutation clearly know that the disease is an eventuality. Many people in these families do not wish to know their genetic status, although some do get tested.

Currently, there is no predictive genetic test for ordinary late-onset Alzheimer's, which is associated with old age. There is one well-defined susceptibility gene, an apolipoprotein E ε4 allele on chromosome 19 (apoE = protein; APOE = gene), which was discovered in 1993 and found to be associated with susceptibility to late-onset Alzheimer's (after fifty-five years of age). A single ε4 gene (found in about one-third of the general population) is not predictive of Alzheimer's in asymptomatic individuals—that is, it does not come close to foretelling whether an individual will eventually have the disease, and many people with the gene never will. Among the 2 percent of people with two of the ε4 genes, however, Alzheimer's might well occur at some point, but there is no indication whatsoever of when, and a person might easily get through a long life with two of these genes and never be affected.

Based on community dialogues in forty-seven state Alzheimer's Association chapters, our NIH-funded guidelines regarding genetic testing were published in the *Journal of the American Medical Association* (Post et al. 1997). Such susceptibility testing can be appropriate in a research setting but is not encouraged in clinical practice because it provides no reliable predictive information upon which to base decisions, it has no medical use, and it may result in discrimination in obtaining disability or long-term care insurance (Post et al. 1997; Alzheimer's Disease Association 2001).

Q11: Should I file a living will or a durable power
of attorney for health care?

A11: A durable power of attorney for health care
is a good idea.

Disclosing a diagnosis of Alzheimer's early in the disease process
allows the person to be involved in communicating and planning for
end-of-life decisions. Diagnostic truth-telling is the necessary starting
point for an ethics of "precedent autonomy" for those who wish to
implement control over their future through advance directives such
as a durable power of attorney for health care, which allows a trusted
loved one to make any and all treatment decisions once the agent
becomes incompetent. This can effectively be coupled with a living
will or some other specific indication of the agent's material wishes
with regard to end-of-life care. Unless the person knows the probable diagnosis in a timely way while still competent to file such legal
instruments, however, the risk that they will be subjected to burdensome medical technologies is increased. Fortunately, many techno-
logically advanced countries now allow next of kin to decide against
efforts to extend life in severe dysfunction, even in the absence of
such legal forms. This is important because numerous patients suffer incapacitating cognitive decline long before having a diagnostic
workup, and even those who are diagnosed early enough to exercise
their autonomy can quickly become incapacitated.

The Alzheimer's Association (2001) asserts that the refusal or
withdrawal of any and all medical treatment is a moral and legal
right for all competent Americans who have reached maturity, and
this right can be asserted by a family surrogate acting on the basis of
either "substituted judgment" (what would the patient when compe-

tent have wanted) or "best interests" (what seems the most humane and least burdensome option at the present time).

The Association concludes that Alzheimer's disease in its advanced stage should be defined as a terminal disease, as roughly delineated by such features as the inability to recognize loved ones, to communicate by speech, to ambulate, or to maintain bowel and/or bladder control. When Alzheimer's progresses to this stage, swallowing difficulties and weight loss will inevitably emerge. Death can be expected for most patients within a year or two, or even sooner, regardless of medical efforts. One useful consequence of viewing the advanced stage as terminal is that family members will better appreciate the importance of palliative care (pain medication) as an alternative to medical treatments intended to extend the dying process. All efforts at life extension in this advanced stage create burdens and avoidable suffering for patients who could otherwise live out the remainder of their lives in greater comfort and peace. Cardiopulmonary resuscitation, dialysis, tube feeding, and all other invasive technologies should be avoided. The use of antibiotics usually does not prolong survival, and comfort can usually be maintained without antibiotic use in patients experiencing infections. Physicians and other health care professionals should recommend this less burdensome and therefore more appropriate approach to family members, and to persons with dementia who are competent, ideally soon after initial diagnosis. Early discussions of a peaceful dying should occur between persons with dementia and their families, guided by information from health care professionals on the relative benefits of a palliative care approach.

Avoiding hospitalization will also decrease the number of persons with advanced Alzheimer's who receive tube feeding, since many long-term care facilities send residents to hospitals for tube placement, after which they return to the facility. It should be remembered that the practice of long-term tube feeding in persons with advanced dementia began only in the mid-1980s after the develop-ment of a new technique called percutaneous endoscopic gastros-tomy (PEG). Before then, such persons were cared for through assisted oral feeding. In comparison with assisted oral feeding, how-ever, long-term tube feeding has no advantages and a number of dis-advantages (Post 2001; Alzheimer's Disease Association 2001).

Q12: Will my remaining ability to make choices be respected?
A12: Hopefully.

People with dementia should be allowed to exercise whatever capaci-ties they retain to make choices and accomplish specific tasks, consis-tent with their independence and dignity.

As discussed in the answer to question 11 above, competent peo-ple have a moral and legal right to reject any medical treatment. Many people with less severe dementia retain this right as well, and it should be protected. People with dementia can find it distressing to have their wishes overridden in areas in which they are still compe-tent, and this situation should be avoided. False accusations of incom-petence can leave an elderly person feeling worthless and hopeless, and even when a person is incompetent in some specific area, care-givers should seek the least restrictive alternative when providing supportive help.

Just as it is obligatory to protect a person with dementia from seriously harmful consequences, it is also obligatory to respect their competent decisions. Diagnosis of Alzheimer's alone is not an indi-cation of incapacity; a person with dementia may lack the mental capacity to drive, handle financial affairs, or live independently in the community but may still be able to make decisions about place of res-idence and medical care.

Concern for the autonomy of people with dementia requires that their capacities be assessed with regard to specific tasks (by means of a "functional assessment"). Determining the locus of power to make decisions rests on this assessment, so it should not be taken lightly. Rather than a single ability that people either possess or lack, competency is defined as a series of abilities, some of which may be present while others are absent.

Conflict arises when the person with dementia insists on doing something that he or she is incompetent to do, failing to recognize the intolerable risks to self or others. In such cases, legal guardianship may be required. For example, a person with dementia who insists on cooking on a gas range, despite having caused one or more fires in their apartment, may require a guardian with the power to determine that person's living situation or even place of residence. Guardianship is an extreme measure, however, which can usually be avoided with good communication and creative intervention. While good care requires an acceptable level of safety, risks should not be exaggerated.

In almost all cases, judgments of an individual's capacity to make medical decisions in a health care setting can be arrived at without the need for legal proceedings. In medical contexts, rough judgments of a patient's specific capacity are routinely made informally by attending physicians, other health care professionals, and family members. Assessment can be straightforward and based on common sense (for example, when an elderly patient is obviously incoherent in conversation, retains little or no information, responds to the same repeated question with seemingly antithetical statements, and lacks insight into the consequences of a decision or its alternatives). There is no justification for protecting an autonomy that the person does not possess.

Capacity, whether clinical or nonclinical, includes the ability to understand relevant options and their consequences in the light of one's own values. In the standard definition of a patient's capacity for medical treatment decision making, an essential element is their ability to understand the nature, purpose, risks, benefits, and alternatives of the proposed treatment. More specifically, a patient needs to be able to: (1) appreciate that he or she has a choice; (2) understand the medical situation and prognosis, the nature of the recommended care, the risks and benefits of each alternative, and the likely consequences; and (3) maintain sufficient decisional stability over time, in contrast to the profound vacillation that indicates an absence of capacity (Lo 1990). Reasonable indecision or changing one's mind does not in and of itself indicate incapacity. During routine conversations, however, a person with advanced dementia can vacillate from one moment to the next in complete self-contradiction, a clear indication of incompetency.

Capacity assessment requires a "sliding scale" (Buchanan and Brock 1990). If a patient refuses a clearly beneficial surgery that promises to restore a better quality of life, a relatively high standard of capacity and measure of certitude would be desired before honoring such a request. If the consequences of a decision are minor, the standards of competence can be lower.

Again, it is important to plan for the global incompetency of advanced dementia through the use of advance directives, especially the durable power of attorney for health care (see question 11 above). To extend one's autonomy prospectively when diagnosed with probable Alzheimer's, estate wills, living wills, and durable powers of attorney for health care are necessary. The precedent self that is fully intact before the clinical manifestation of dementia has the legal right and authority to dictate levels of medical care for the severely demented self. Questions can arise about the capacity of the precedent self to make these decisions, since he or she has not experienced the demented state and may view it too negatively. The fact remains, however, that legally the right to determine treatment limitations is established by advance directive legislation.

Q13: Will I be physically or chemically restrained?
A13: Hopefully not.

The best approach to problem behaviors relies on social and environmental modifications and creative activities, thereby preserving the individual's independence and self-esteem. Activities that creatively draw on their remaining abilities, coupled with adaptive changes in their immediate surroundings and in how others interact with them, can positively influence the behavior of people with dementia. Art and music programs, for example, are often helpful in refocusing their attention and energies. In dealing with agitated behavior, health professionals and family members should always try to establish a calm environment with soft music and lighting, approach the agitated person slowly and calmly, speak in a reassuring and gentle tone of voice, use a gentle touch, maintain nonthreatening postures, and avoid arguing.

Wandering is a behavior that occurs in up to 26 percent of nursing home residents and up to 59 percent of people with dementia who still live at home (Cohen-Mansfield et al. 1991). Many people with dementia will never wander; among those who do, however, wandering can occur unexpectedly. It is important to consider what might be causing the wandering—for example, changes in environment, disturbing noises, restlessness, anxiety, overmedication leading to mental confusion, physical need, or sometimes even searching for a real or imagined object. Some studies suggest that wandering should be encouraged as a person's way of coping with stress, especially for those who, before the onset of Alzheimer's, responded to stress by engaging in physical activities such as pacing (Algase 1992).

As much as possible, people with dementia should remain free to wander in areas that are hazard-free and nonthreatening. Involuntary restraint is unethical and illegal, and because of various side effects there is no current drug therapy for wandering that will not also potentially interfere with other valued activities. Therefore, caregivers should view wandering as beneficial to the affected individual and look for creative ways to allow it to occur in a safe, protective environment, such as modifications to the immediate surroundings. The Alzheimer's Association now also has a Safe Return program, a nationwide registry of people with Alzheimer's that provides each individual with an identity bracelet or necklace.

Physical and chemical restraints should not be substituted for social, environmental, and activity modifications. Physical restraints result in unnecessary immobility and are frequently hazardous: for example, people with dementia struggle for freedom and can harm themselves in the process. Strangulation, medical ailments caused by immobility, and increased agitation are among the serious and substantial harms caused by physical restraints (Johnson 1990). Concern for the safety of the person with dementia is significant, especially because for the frail elderly falls can be very serious. But the potential harms of physical restraints must also be counted as risks to safety. Moreover, physical restraints increase the Alzheimer's-affected person's perception of threat (Patel and Hope 1993). Their use is partly the result of fear of lawsuits against nursing homes, although such suits are rare. While safety is important, it does not justify involuntary restraint and the indignity of being tied down.

Health professionals need to be attentive to how family caregivers control the behavior of individuals with Alzheimer's and should encourage individualized and diverse approaches that do not resort to chemical and physical restraints (Reifler, Henry, and Sherrill 1992). However, family caregivers may pressure physicians to "do something" quickly about behaviors that are offensive or frightening and cause emotional stress in the family. Society has come to expect prompt control of such behaviors, even if control requires resorting to chemical means. If caregivers are already "women in the middle" dealing with many competing obligations, an aging parent in a delusional or agitated state can be the last straw. For these and other reasons, some of them economic, it can be difficult for family members to sustain a commitment to using only environmental and psychosocial methods of behavioral control, although these are preferable to medication for most behavioral problems. In such circumstances, families may need to rely on pharmacology to a greater extent than they might otherwise have done.

Ideally, efforts to change the physical or psychosocial environment should be tried before drugs are prescribed. If caregivers must resort to behavior-controlling drugs, however, they should be used cautiously and only for specified purposes. If psychoactive drugs are used, the purpose of treatment and the target symptom must be well defined; as few drugs as possible should be used, and they should be administered starting with low doses, increasing dosages slowly and monitoring carefully for side effects (Martin and Whitehouse 1990).

Taking multiple medications concurrently for the same condition, as well as overmedication, are particular problems in the dementia patient population. Both clinical experience and scientific evidence indicate that patients' behavior can be controlled at lower dosages than are commonly given. Moreover, drugs to reduce disturbed behaviors (such as wandering, restlessness, irritability) create ethical issues when used at doses that interfere with a patient's remaining cognitive function and cause other side effects.

Used sparingly in this context, drugs can have the desired therapeutic effects, which also help to maintain the home care environment, lighten the burden on caregivers, and make the use of physical restraints unnecessary. Thus, when used carefully to attain defined short-term goals, drugs can be highly beneficial, making caregiving more manageable without compromising the person's quality of life.

Q14: Can I drive?

A14: For a while, but there will come a time to stop rather than risk causing harm.

Eventually, everyone with a worsening dementia will need to stop driving—something that clinicians should address up front because there is so much primacy and authority in their position. A visit or two after a diagnosis of probable Alzheimer's is made, clinicians need to ask: "Do you drive and does it mean a lot to you?" Begin the conversation with the central family caregiver in the room. The conversation will unfold differently for each case, and the clinician can offer any help through a clinical social worker or other support. Sometimes this conversation unfolds well over the months ahead, but the caregiver needs to know they can ask the clinician for help if things get dangerous and their loved one insists on driving. Ideally, the affected individual can come to be involved in this monumental decision. Family members and the affected person must know that if an accident occurs that injures others, the family may be held financially liable and insurers may not be obliged to cover this liability.

In many cases, the person's autonomy and self-perception are threatened by limits on driving. Especially in cultural traditions that emphasize independence and control, relying on others for transportation can be perceived as demeaning. Moreover, driving can have tremendous significance as a symbol of individual freedom, and limitations can be an unwelcome sign of dependence.

A diagnosis of Alzheimer's is never itself sufficient reason for loss of driving privileges. Individuals with Alzheimer's are at risk for driving impairments; if they are actually impaired, privileges must be limited for the sake of public safety. Eventually all people with progressive dementia must stop driving when they become a serious risk to self or others.

Individuals are often capable of driving for several years or more after diagnosis, depending on when the diagnosis is made and on the rate of disease progression. Partial limits can be designed for the individual who may be able to drive safely in familiar surroundings, in daylight, or in good weather. Although there is an indisputable duty to prevent people from driving if they clearly threaten community safety, this principle should not be applied prematurely or without an individualized risk appraisal that clearly demonstrates impairment of driving ability.

Whether the physician or other health professionals should have a central role in the restriction of driving privileges remains unclear; but the physician should be willing to play a part as needed. In situations where the family simply cannot negotiate limits on driving with a loved one who is a danger to self and others, it behooves the clinician to recommend firmly to the individual that their driving be limited or halted entirely. This technique will usually succeed. If not, the family may need to hide the car keys or even disable any vehicles as a last resort.

I do not support mandatory reporting of a probable diagnosis of Alzheimer's to the Department of Motor Vehicles. There are a number of reasons for my position, one of which is that mandatory physician reporting singles out people with dementia and violates their right to confidentiality. In addition, reporting requirements might discourage some persons from coming to see their doctor for diagnosis early in the course of disease, when drug treatments are most clearly indicated. California is one state that does mandate physician reporting of people with Alzheimer's, and the information is forwarded to the Department of Motor Vehicles. The person is then required to be assessed for driving abilities (State of California 1987). This approach frees physicians and families from a fear of lawsuits (should the patient have an accident) and the need to make a risk assessment.

The person with dementia, if competent, should participate in decision making regarding driving restrictions. Appropriate limits to driving and other activities of daily living can often be delineated and mutually agreed upon through open communication among the affected person, family, and health care professionals. Individual responses to proposed limits can vary from immediate acceptance to strong resistance; to encourage acceptance, the individual who agrees to limits should be assured that others, such as family members, will assist in providing transportation. Indeed, in discussions of limits related to dementia, family members can often avoid conflict with the affected individual by identifying and supplying alternatives to risky activities, including driving.

Ideally, however, a privilege is never limited without offering the person ways to compensate and lessen any sense of loss. An "all or nothing" approach can and should be avoided, and the affected person should be a major participant in negotiations and retain a sense of freedom and self-control, if possible (Alzheimer's Disease Association 2001). Compromise and adjustments can be successfully implemented by those who are informed and caring, especially when the person with Alzheimer's has insight into his or her diminishing mental abilities and loss of competence. The Alzheimer's-affected person who lacks insight into the consequences of the disease, of course, is more likely to refuse to stop driving, resulting in the need to impose restrictions that may be resisted.

Necessary restrictions on daily activities besides driving also have a great deal of significance for many people with dementia. For example, a person may need to avoid street crossings while out for walks alone if they forget that a green light means proceed. Cooking privileges are another example. A gradual, caring, negotiated approach to restrictions is best, protecting privileges and freedoms as much as possible while making efforts to substitute other valued activities for the ones that are lost. The lives of people with dementia should be as free and fulfilling as possible; a totally safe, risk-free existence is neither possible nor beneficial.

A key rule is always this: "Never a no without a yes." For example, "Now you cannot drive any more, but we will take you out wherever you want to go. Just let us know."

Q15: Should I participate in research?

A15: You can, but you don't need to.

Regarding research consent, a deeply forgetful person who still has the capacity to make decisions for research can do so if the research is minimal risk, regardless of whether there is any potential benefit for self. If there is some potential risk, the individual with capacity can also consent for research regardless of whether there is any likely benefit for self. However, once that person loses capacity, and can therefore no longer decide to withdraw from the research for whatever reason, then research can only continue if a surrogate (usually the caregiver) provides consent and the research has some possible therapeutic value for the subject. A surrogate can consent for an affected individual when that individual lacks decision-making ability if the risks are minimal (regardless of whether the research is purely

altruistic or has potential benefits to the subject), or if there are significant risks, but the potential therapeutic benefits are reasonably
apparent. No, a surrogate cannot volunteer an affected individual for
risky research that has no likely benefit to that subject.

In 2001 I helped the Alzheimer's Association draft a statement
addressing when proxy or surrogate consent was allowable with
respect to risk and benefits. It concluded that:

a. For minimal risk research all individuals should be allowed
   to enroll, even if there is no potential benefit to the individual. In the absence of an advance directive, proxy consent is
   acceptable.

b. For greater than minimal risk research *and* if there is a reasonable potential for benefit to the individual, the enrollment of
   all individuals with Alzheimer disease is allowable based on
   proxy consent. The proxy's consent can be based on either a
   research specific advance directive *or* the proxy's judgment of
   the individual's best interests.

c. For greater than minimal risk research *and* if there is *no* reasonable potential for benefit to the individual only those individuals who (1) are capable of giving their own informed consent, or (2) have executed a research specific advance directive
   are allowed to participate. In either case, a proxy must be
   available to monitor the individual's involvement in the
   research. (Note: this provision means that individuals who
   are not capable of making their own decisions about research
   participation and have not executed an advance directive or
   do not have a proxy to monitor their participation cannot participate in this category of research.)

The Association indicates that surrogates must not allow their hopes
for effective therapies to overtake their critical assessment of the
facts, or to diminish the significance of participant expressions of
dissent. Subject dissent or other expressions of agitation should be

respected, although a surrogate can attempt reasonable levels of persuasion or assistance. People with dementia, for example, may initially refuse to have blood drawn or to take medication; once a family member helps calm the situation and explain things, they may change their minds. This kind of assistance is acceptable. Continued dissent, however, requires withdrawal of the participant from the study, even if surrogates would prefer to see the research participation continue.

To date, so much research on deeply forgetful people has been biomedical—in search of an effective drug—but this search has as yet been largely fruitless. It may just be that, as Dr. Alzheimer himself thought, senility is simply a part of brain aging and we are not likely to fix it. Thus, we need to learn how to accept it and use our research dollars instead on psychosocial interventions, on better assisted living facilities like those in Denmark, which enjoy wide popularity, and on supporting caregivers both in the home and in the nursing home. While biomedical research is welcome, it has received the largest share of funding but has not yielded much in the way of concrete results, while we have failed to fully and deeply explore all the nonbiological interventions that can do so much more for deeply forgetful people and their caregivers without in any way subjecting them to physical or mental risks, discomfort, or pain.

Q16: Can I avoid technology and tubes so I can just die naturally?

A16: Yes, avoid medical technology, including artificial nutrition and hydration of any kind.

One useful consequence of viewing the advanced stage of Alzheimer's as terminal is that family members will better appreciate the importance of palliative care (pain medication) as an alternative to medical treatments intended to extend the dying process. All efforts at life extension in this advanced stage create burdens and avoidable suffering for patients who could otherwise live out the remainder of their lives in greater comfort and peace. Cardiopulmonary resuscitation, dialysis, tube feeding, and all other invasive technologies should be avoided. Physicians and other health care professionals should recommend this less burdensome and therefore more appropriate approach to family members, and to persons with dementia who are competent, ideally soon after initial diagnosis. Early discussions of a peaceful dying should occur between persons with dementia and their families, guided by information from health care professionals on the relative benefits of a palliative care approach.

Deeply forgetful people are always present underneath the chaos or the silence, and they always possess consciousness as they take in the world around them. The fact that their rational processes are disordered or even absent is irrelevant with regard to the respect they are owed as members of the human family. We need to keep in mind that they can have relatively good days as well as bad ones, and that this is the only life they have. The quality of their lives depends largely on those of us who recognize how we can help them and, in the process, help ourselves as we gain insights into the ways and the power of love to reveal the continuities of selfhood. On my visits to her as a child my grandma was always there, although quietly so, and I personally believe that she now rests—fully herself—in the hands of the Infinite.

But we ought not to stretch out the lives of deeply forgetful people with the use of any medical technologies whatsoever. As I have made clear, we need not continue to treat diabetes, heart failure, kidney failure, or any form of cancer, except perhaps to perform surgery for purely palliative reasons. Lung intubation, nasogastric tubes, dialysis, PEG feeding, resuscitation, and any and all of the life-extending technologies used in hospitals these days are simply blatant forms of torture imposed on quiet souls who are ready to move on from this world.

In the 1990s, when feeding PEGs were displacing assisted oral feeding in nursing homes, I was able to convince many adult children that once a deeply forgetful person stops swallowing, it is nature's way of providing them with the gift of a peaceful death through the release of the body's natural opioid-like chemicals, the endorphins. This is true not just with Alzheimer's, but with cancer and literally every major disease: the gastrointestinal system naturally shuts down, and palliative chemicals (endorphins) are released from the brain in the absence of food and water.

To this day, though, I see deeply forgetful people stuck with every sort of needle and device in hospitals and sometimes even in unenlightened nursing homes, and I cringe. Not long ago I heard an old woman in such a situation moaning all day and even crying out "Help" from time to time. Her family just did not understand how much suffering they were causing in attempting to honor the value of life. Fortunately, I was able to speak with them later in her room as I was visiting during clinical pastoral care rounds and convinced them that what they were doing had to stop.

There ought to be a public policy rule against any and all technological violation of deeply forgetful people. Such suffering is ethically and spiritually obscene. When they reach the end of life, many people have not prepared an advance directive, they have not created a durable power of attorney to deal with health care decisions, and their poor family members feel guilty if they don't summon all the marvels of modern medical technology to treat them. So that their wishes might be carried out in the final stages of the disease, preventing discomfort and a loss of dignity, patients with Alzheimer's need to do both of these things, as I have emphasized—leave advance directives and assign someone the durable power of attorney. Taking these steps reassures those diagnosed with Alzheimer's that they will not have their lives extended in the grip of an unwanted technological imperative.

The goal that I have tried to convince families of is this: in almost all cases palliative care alone is preferred. Patients in the advanced stage of dementia are often subjected to invasive procedures including CPR, treatment for diabetes, continued treatment for heart failure, and even tube feeding when little clinical benefit is to be expected. Of course, any pain should be treated with pain medications—including antibiotics for urinary and other painful infections, and in some cases for lung infections. There are also some good drugs for behavioral problems that cannot be managed environmentally.

Because of the difficulties inherent in caring for a patient with advanced dementia, 90 percent of Americans with dementia will be institutionalized before death. Many deeply forgetful people are transferred out of the nursing home into acute-care hospitals at various points, where invasive procedures are readily performed (Mitchell 2004). In addition, because Alzheimer's is not considered a terminal illness—although it should be—at the last assessment before death only half of dementia patients had an advance directive in place to limit invasive care, but over 85 percent of cancer patients did. This discrepancy is reflected in the fact that five times more dementia patients than cancer patients were subjected to an invasive treatment such as tube feeding, in part because professionals and family do not clearly acknowledge that such patients are terminally ill (McNamara and Kennedy 2001).

Research has shown that patients' quality of life in the terminal stages of dementia is not at the acceptable level that families and physicians should attempt to provide for them. Patients with advanced

dementia do experience symptoms at the end of life that are responsive to palliative care, such as constipation and pain, yet health care
workers often fail to treat these symptoms in a manner that provides
relief. Instead, patients with dementia actually have more markers
associated with poor quality of nursing home care, such as pressure
ulcers, the use of restraints, and the use of antipsychotic medications,
than do patients with cancer (Mitchell 2004). It is possible that, in the
patients with dementia, the medication and restraints may be used
to control agitation that is actually a result of unmanaged pain. But
restraints are uncomfortable and potentially dangerous to elderly
patients, and do not promote palliation in any way. Clearly an accurate assessment of their individual needs, followed by proper palliative treatment, would be of great benefit to these patients.

Patients with dementia also benefit from the palliative care provided by hospice programs much less often than do patients with
cancer and other terminal illnesses (Mendiratta et al. 2003). Alzheimer's patients are less likely to be transferred to hospice because it
is difficult to predict their survival time, and a referral to hospice
requires that death be expected to occur within six months (Mitchell 2004). However, in many nursing homes today, visiting hospice
teams have made great progress in influencing the prevailing culture
and practices, and providing hospice-style care in nursing homes
is much better than transferring a deeply forgetful person to a hospice where staff may not be well trained in managing these patients.
Home hospice care is, of course, also recommended.

Please No Tubes, Just the
Old-Fashioned Assisted Oral Feeding

In the mid-1980s and throughout the 1990s (Hanson, Garrett, and
Lewis 2008), gastrostomy tube feeding became commonplace in
patients with advanced dementia and in elderly patients more gen-

erally, following the development of the PEG procedure. This relatively simple procedure passes a feeding tube directly through the nearby skin and then into the stomach, a procedure thought to be a humane way to keep patients adequately fed and hydrated. Hanson, Garrett, and Lewis show how physicians hoped that PEG tube placement would reduce associated complications, such as bedsores resulting from malnutrition or aspiration pneumonia.

The PEG procedure was developed by my former colleague, Dr. Michael Gauderer, at Rainbow Babies and Children's Hospital in Cleveland (1979–1980), for use in young children with swallowing difficulties. The procedure required only local anesthesia, thus eliminating the significant surgical risk associated with general anesthesia and infection (Gauderer and Ponsky 1981). Gauderer wrote two decades later that while PEG use has benefited countless patients, "in part because of its simplicity and low complication rate, this minimally invasive procedure also lends itself to over-utilization" (Gauderer 1999, 883). Expressing moral concerns about the proliferation of the procedure, Gauderer indicated that as the third decade of PEG use began to unfold, "much of our effort in the future needs to be directed toward ethical aspects" (Gauderer 1999, 882). At present, PEG is being used more frequently even in those patients for whom these procedures were deemed too risky in the past.

For more than two decades researchers have underscored the burdens and risks of PEG tube feeding in persons with advanced dementia. The growing literature was well summarized in a review by Finucane, Christmas, and Travis, who found no published evidence that tube feeding prevents aspiration pneumonia, prolongs survival, reduces the risks of pressure sores or infections, improves function, or provides palliation in this population (Finucane, Christmas, and Travis 1999; Gillick 2000; Post 2001).

PEG use is not really "easy," due to its technological complexities, and the recipient will usually develop diarrhea. In some cases, physical restraints are used to keep a person from pulling on the several inches of tube that extend out of the abdomen. One wonders if assisted oral feeding is not easier after all. Regardless, supposed technical ease and efficiency do not mean that these technologies should be utilized. Should persons with advanced progressive dementia ever be provided with PEGs? In general, assisted oral feeding and hospice are better alternatives than tube feeding, although there will be some cases where the limited capacities of an informal family caregiver justify it as the ethically necessary alternative to starvation when the patient's ability to swallow has begun to diminish. Ideally, home health aides would make assisted oral feeding possible even in these cases, but this is not a priority in our current health care system. Institutions, however, should uniformly provide assisted oral feeding as the preferred alternative to tube feeding, a measure that would profoundly obviate the overuse of this technology.

Physicians and other health care professionals should recommend a less burdensome and therefore more appropriate approach to family members, and to persons with dementia who are competent, ideally soon after initial diagnosis, although not all physicians agree with this view (Teno, Meltzer, and Mitchell 2014). Persons with dementia and their families should discuss a peaceful dying early in the course of the disease, guided by information from health care professionals on the relative benefits of a palliative care approach, and emphasizing assisted oral feeding (Zapka, Amella, and Magwood 2014; Volicer and Hurley 1998).

Early in the course of Alzheimer's, individuals may manifest irregular feeding patterns; as dementia progresses, however, they eventually lose the capacity to swallow both solids and liquids (Mitchell, Teno, and Kiely 2009). For family members, the subsequent weight loss can be ethically and emotionally challenging and can result in requests that the individual receive artificial nutrition and hydration. There is also some tendency to want to insist on PEG feeding in non-Caucasians, mainly as a response to historical injustice that, while meaningful, has not been shown to benefit the patient (Braun, Rabeneck, and McCullough 2005).

In the late 1990s clinical research emerged that questioned the benefits of PEG tubes in advanced dementia. Several studies (Meier, Ahronheim, and Morris 2001; Teno, Gozalo, and Mitchell 2012a; Teno, Gozalo, and Mitchell 2012b) showed that the supposed benefits of PEG feeding (decreased aspiration pneumonia, decreased pressure ulcers with improved nutrition, increased survival) were nonexistent when compared to hand feeding (assisted oral feeding) by a caregiver. Gillick (2000) concluded that when the potential disadvantages of PEG use (increased chemical/physical restraints on patients, lack of gustatory pleasure and caregiver bonding) are considered, PEG must be judged non-beneficial.

Here are some standard items to use in assisted feeding for a person with Alzheimer's in that final year or months.

Recipes

When it is difficult to get the patient to eat enough, make every bite count. These are some ideas—be creative.

JUICY GELATIN

1 package gelatin	Prepare gelatin as usual, except
1 cup hot water	substitute juice for the cold water.
1 cup fruit juice	

MILKY GELATIN

....

1 package gelatin	Prepare gelatin as usual, except
1 cup hot water	substitute milk for the cold water.
1 cup fruit milk	

APPLESAUCE PRUNE BRAN

....

½ cup bran	Mix together and serve 2 table-
½ cup prune juice	spoons with each meal. (Do not
½ cup applesauce	give to patients with poor intake
	of fluids.)

Cervo, Bryan, and Farber (2006) describe family disputes and mis-aligned expectations that can pressure physicians into providing PEG feeding despite a patient's advance directives to the contrary. I have served on three ethics panels (Post 2001 and the American Geriatrics Society Ethics Committee and Clinical Practice and Models of Care Committee [AGS] 2014), all of which recommended against PEG use (the American Geriatrics Society and the Alzheimer's Associations of the United States and Canada) and instead urged acceptance of late Alzheimer's disease as a terminal illness for which hand feeding and comfort care are appropriate. This recommendation aligns with the preferences of most elderly Americans; one study (American Geriatrics Society 2014) found that of older adult respondents (aged sixty-five-plus) who are cognitively intact, fewer than one in twenty would want tube feeding or CPR in late-stage dementia.

Despite the trend away from this procedure in the early 2000s (Teno, Mitchell, and Gozalo 2010), many geriatricians and ethicists continue to note instances (Schulze, Mazzola, and Hoffman 2016) of unnecessary PEG tube placements in patients with advanced dementia. Several studies (Bell, Somogyi-Zalud, and Masaki 2008; Komiya, Ishii, and Teramoto 2012; Nakanishi and Hattor 2014; Schulze, Mazzola, and Hoffman 2016) indicate that in the United States and other medically advanced nations, PEG use still remains the default option in many regions and states.

Avoiding hospitalization will help decrease the number of persons with advanced Alzheimer's who receive tube feeding, since many long-term care facilities send residents to hospitals for tube placement, after which they return to the facility. It should be remembered that the practice of long-term tube feeding in persons with advanced dementia began only in the mid-1980s after the development of a new technique called percutaneous endoscopic gastrostomy (PEG). Before then, such persons were cared for through assisted oral feeding. As noted earlier, though, in comparison with assisted oral feeding, long-term tube feeding has no advantages, and a number of disadvantages (Alzheimer's Disease Association 2001).

Conclusions

In conclusion, it is wise for deeply forgetful people to avoid medical technologies, especially PEG feeding, ventilators, dialysis, cardiac devices, resuscitation, surgery, and the like. So how can technology help them? Just as we see countless devices populating the lives of those who are supposedly memory "intact," there are today all sorts of "assistive technologies" for deeply forgetful people, and these technologies can help ease anxiety, establish routines, improve quality of life, and promote autonomy and independence. Special clocks, picture-adapted telephones, devices for monitoring electrical appliance use, GPS tracking, home care robots, reminder texts and messages, and lots of other innovative gadgets can be useful. This is an emerging field that is going to become more and more important in the care of people with Alzheimer's. We may eventually see memory chips implanted into the brain, or brains hooked up directly to computers. It is possible that the use of new devices will be much more beneficial than any of the existing purportedly memory-enhancing drugs, none of which actually do much of anything. Perhaps the evolution of memory-enhancing technology will encourage greater respect for deeply forgetful people, who are increasingly dependent, like the rest of us, on devices galore.

4

The Seventeenth Question:
Preemptive Physician-Assisted Suicide (PPAS) for Alzheimer's Disease

A Caution

Any progressive neurological condition is a hard thing for anyone to confront. Though multiple sclerosis, Parkinson's disease, Lou Gehrig's disease, Alzheimer's disease, chronic traumatic encephalopathy, and others are all different from one another, these conditions can for some raise the biggest question: "to be, or not to be."

I have coined the term "preemptive physician-assisted suicide" (PPAS) to designate a request for assisted suicide by a person who is still lucid of mind, who knows that they face a severe cognitive decline in the years ahead, and who would like to "preempt" such a decline by availing themselves of physician-assisted suicide while they are still able to do so. This occurs in such places as the Netherlands and Switzerland. PPAS is not "euthanasia" (being killed by someone other than self) but suicide in the sense that a physician would typically prescribe enough barbiturates for the individual to mix in a thick drink such as a milkshake and swallow. Because this is illegal in the United States, the physician would leave the patient and family or friend to perform this ritual of self-termination on their own. I do not advocate for this practice, but neither have I wished to criticize any of the several dozen individuals I have encountered over the years who have in fact determined to take their lives rather than experience a decline that they viewed as a fate worse than death.

Two Cases of PPAS

My experience with PPAS goes back many years. As a doctoral student at the University of Chicago in the early 1980s, I knew two famed psychiatrists diagnosed with probable Alzheimer's, and both were mentors. One, Dr. K., had a loving family and spent the next decade in an impressive nursing home in Hyde Park; the other, Dr. B., swallowed a milky concoction of forty Seconal tablets, went to bed, and never woke up. Dr. B. had no family or any sort of support network, nor did he wish to depend on home health aides. He was not depressed, but as a gifted scholar he refused to allow his capacity for thought and related scholarly activity to fade. Since he was a psychiatrist, he was able to get all the capsules he needed. In contrast to Dr. K., who enjoyed the love and support of a wonderful family, Dr. B. was what we now hear referred to as a "live alone" and had none of these assets.

In 1999, a year when I received the Jennifer B. Langston Community Service Award from the Cleveland-area chapter of the Alzheimer's Association, I was speaking with two families in which a person in the early phase of deep forgetfulness had, with familial support, developed plans for assisted suicide. In neither case did I condone these plans, and I recommended against PPAS because I felt that there was a better way forward. But in both cases the individual affected by Alzheimer's was capable, determined, and had family support that only grew firmer with time.

I recognized at the time that when an individual has firmly set-tled on PPAS and cannot be dissuaded, I could still be present and alongside them without being complicit or feeling compromised. So, I have been a gentle witness rather than a helper, and I have said prayers with some individuals diagnosed with Alzheimer's and their families in peaceful home settings as they prepared to die by their own hand while they still could lift a glass filled with carefully pre-pared liquid.

Such events as I have witnessed them are not gruesome but rather are quite serene; they are not the result of despair but rather of hope understood as an alternative to gradual decline; and they are not the result of depression, but rather have been matters of rational choice based on a burden-versus-benefit analysis, subjectively considered.

Grandma J

In a stately old home in a Cleveland suburb Grandma J was still very clearheaded and making everyday decisions. She had made up her own mind about things from very early in life, and even had a per-sonal motto: "More defiant than reliant." But she was slowly losing her ability to read with comprehension, and she had always been an avid reader. She could no longer play her violin. She had three grand-children, but they were grown up now and had so much respect for Grandma J that they were not willing to question her resolve. Over a period of five months Grandma J and I spoke five times over after-noon tea, and each time she grew firmer in her resolve. I was clear that I felt she still had a lot to offer the world and her family, but her constant refrain was to assert her self-reliance. We talked about inter-dependence and the way human beings all depend on one another, especially in times of illness or decline, and I said that this can be a deeply meaningful and even fulfilling experience of affirmation and care. But I did not make the slightest dent in her willful decision. The next time we spoke, she said, "Goodbye now, but I will call you." About a week later, I received a call from Grandma J inviting me over on Sunday evening for her "final exit." I did not decline, but I responded with hope that she might still see things differently. As the week passed, I decided to make this 5 p.m. rendezvous and to at least be there with respectful and affective presence. I rang the bell and her son let me in. There was Grandma J sitting by the big brick fireplace talking quietly with her two adult children who were about my age and one granddaughter who especially loved her and wanted very much to be present. There next to Grandma J's chair was a table upon which I could see a large colorful teacup, the one she seemed always to like. She was comfortable by the fireplace, watching the flames dart about and feeling pleasantly warm.

"We are like the fire, each one of us a flame flickering in the whole. We are a part of something so much greater than we are individually. I am leaving some wonderful things behind while I still can and so I don't get trapped. Now let us pray."

And she prayed aloud. With her daughter, her son, and her young adult granddaughter there (her beloved husband had passed away years ago), she asked me to say a brief prayer, which I did. Importantly, none of the younger grandchildren were present because they should not have to witness such an event. Peaceful Bach choral music was playing. Everyone spoke about how grateful they were for her life, and she too spoke of how fulfilling and meaningful her life had been, and of how she did not want anyone to think that she wasn't "all in" with her decision. We talked for half an hour or so. The mood was not mirthful, but it was kindly and tranquil. Then Grandma J quickly placed a straw in her mouth and drank the potion down in a minute. After she drank, everyone shared hugs with her, and her son read poems by Robert Frost. As the fire burned brightly she began, after twenty minutes, to fade. Her last words were "More defiant than reliant, but I love you all." Then her eyes closed for good. It was all quite spiritual, profoundly respectful, and entirely gentle throughout.

I left her home about 7 p.m. after saying goodbye to her family members and seeing that they were sad but not distressed. How they managed the details I have no idea, but the local paper wrote in a brief obituary several days later that she had simply died peacefully in her sleep. I of course had very mixed thoughts and feelings about this episode, and it has always stayed with me. Much of what follows in this chapter reflects that deep ambivalence. I did not criticize Grandma J, and I honored her convictions, but I did not see her action as something to celebrate. She did not want to experience any more decline and could see no good reason to endure inevitable losses of self-reliance. Her physician had written a prescription for Grandma J—or perhaps it was a nurse practitioner: I did not know and did not inquire.

Janet Adkins and Dr. Kevorkian

We turn now to the 1990 case that many people are aware of, Michigan pathologist Jack Kevorkian's assisted suicide of Janet Adkins, a fifty-four-year-old member of the Hemlock Society diagnosed with probable Alzheimer's disease. Shortly after the case appeared in newspapers nationwide, Kevorkian applied for a position in our ethics center at Case Western Reserve School of Medicine. My colleagues and I did not invite him in for an interview as he was not academically qualified for the position. In 1998 the Alzheimer's Association national newsletter, *Advances*, published this letter from Ron Adkins, Janet's husband:

My wife, Janet Adkins, was excited by life. She was a woman of many ideas and interests. She was a talented musician and an avid reader. She liked pushing the limit and trying new things, such as trekking through Nepal.

When she was diagnosed with Alzheimer's disease at age 53, she was devastated. She weighed the options of letting the disease take her mind and body or exiting early with the assistance of a doctor while her intellect was still intact. We had openly discussed end-of-life issues, and her choice was not to let the disease progress. Janet hired a therapist to facilitate discussion among family members about her choice. Our three sons respected her decision only after she participated in a drug study that produced no results and no other medical options were available to Janet.

For several months, we exchanged communication and medical information with Dr. Jack Kevorkian. Kevorkian informed us he would assist us, but that the procedure would have to take place in his old rusty Volkswagen van. Janet's response was, "I don't care where I die, I care how I die."

Her death took place just one year after she was diagnosed. I spoke to the media only after the point where they began depicting Janet as a person who was depressed and out of her mind. In her last days, Janet's intellect was still intact and she died with the dignity she desired.

Janet felt so awful that people with a terminal illness can't make a choice to go out with dignity. If she could have signed a legal document that said, "at this point, I want you to end my life," she could have lived an extra year or two with the cognitive life she wanted. But she didn't have that choice.

We made an informed decision and a personal choice, one that was right for Janet. Most importantly we openly discussed end-of-life issues together as a family. I encourage others to do the same.

(Adkins 1998, 2)

Janet Adkins was enrolled in a drug trial for tacrine, the early cholinesterase inhibitor, at the University of Washington's Alzheimer's
Research Center. Like others, she experienced no meaningful or lasting symptomatic benefits. Physicians involved with her treatment
coauthored an article about her case several years after the suicide
occurred (Rohde, Peskind, and Raskind 1995). They described insidi-
ous memory impairment, including word-finding difficulties, which
made it impossible for her to continue her career as a teacher and her
avocation as a pianist. She did, however, still play competitive tennis
and enjoy her family, including grandchildren. She was in good physical health and had no depression. Her local physician informed her
that her disease would progress very rapidly and that she would lose
the capacity for self-care within a year. At the University of Washington during her initial examination, with her husband present, she
stated that she would consider suicide if the drug did not prove beneficial (both she and her husband were members of the Hemlock Society). The physicians told the Adkinses that they did not agree with
the prognosis she had received locally, and that she would not progress to advanced Alzheimer's for two to three years.

Janet did not show any response to the drug, declined further follow-up, and pursued Kevorkian's services despite the Washington
physicians' efforts to encourage counseling. She was confirmed with
a diagnosis of Alzheimer's at autopsy after her assisted suicide.

Sources of Ambivalence:
Five Reasons to Question PPAS

On the face of it, PPAS has a certain hypercognitive (Post 1995b) at-
traction that can only be taken seriously. Many people believe

strongly that if there is one good justification for suicide, Alzheimer's is it. Based on at least twenty informal, unscientific polls I have taken at caregiver conferences, about a third of caregivers are very much against PPAS, another third are in favor of it, and another third are uncertain.

In those few countries where PPAS is legal, such as the Netherlands and Sweden, only about 5 percent of those individuals newly diagnosed with Alzheimer's and thus still able to act autonomously seek this final solution (Tomlinson 2015). These are countries where long-term care and caregiver support systems are very well-subsidized by the governments, a fact that may partly explain why PPAS is not more widely desired. After all, long-term care does not force a couple into spend-down poverty, and respite is well supplied.

The low 5 percent figure is also likely the result of people becoming so deeply forgetful that they no longer remember having any wish for PPAS. The temporal window for PPAS will eventually close because it requires an individual who is competent to act. Perhaps their families and physicians are "waiting them out" until they literally forget that they wanted to preempt Alzheimer's. Or perhaps in some cases they begin to realize that although they are forgetful and increasingly dependent on the kindness of others, this is the one life they have and self-reliance has its limits. I had hoped that Grandma J would have come to this recognition, but she did not.

Let no one judge those who have made their "final exit" through PPAS. Even where it is not legal, this practice goes on quietly, away from the public eye, at least to some degree. In states like Oregon and Washington, where physician-assisted suicide has long been legal for those within an estimated six months of dying, those with a progressive Alzheimer's are clearly excluded because by the time they are that close to dying they will have been incapable of making any rational decision for years.

**Q: REASON ONE: Do you know how this
disease will progress?**

A: Almost never.

It is worth noting that a diagnosis of Alzheimer's is always only probable, especially early on. Many cases are not as progressive (worsening over time) as might be supposed because the Alzheimer's is
"mixed" or in combination with vascular dementia, which is generally not progressive but rather stable. Also, brain, environment, and
social support do interact to a significant degree, meaning that the
progression of Alzheimer's is partly determined by social and external factors (Devi 2017). No two cases follow the same precise course.
For almost all cases, there is no predictive autosomal-dominant and
causative gene that lets anyone know what their fate actually is with
great clarity. So PPAS assumes a still somewhat questionable diagnosis of probable Alzheimer's in the early stage while one remains capable of autonomous acts, and it is very hard to predict the details of
one's future experience, which can be quite varied.

I wondered how long Grandma J would have had a plausibly
good quality of life had she not orchestrated her PPAS. It might have
been years of time with her grandchildren nearby, being inspired by
reading to them as occurs in the various intergenerational schools
around the United States. Maybe she could have gotten an Alzheimer's dog and been overjoyed. How many recorded books might she
have enjoyed? What about listening to all of Bach, and the Cleveland
Orchestra?

This ambiguity about the future trajectory and timing of decline
is nearly universal for people diagnosed with Alzheimer's. However,
there are the rare cases (2 to 3 percent of the total) that are caused
by the autosomal-dominant genes Presenilin 1 or 2 that, if tested,

do allow one to know when Alzheimer's will strike (usually about age forty), that it will run its course relatively quickly over about five years, until death, and that it is a certainty. These early-onset families know their history well. Some were adolescents when their mother or father experienced the ordeal of early-onset disease, and they witnessed the aggressive decline that followed and its impact on their family. If they want to orchestrate their own final exit before their genetically certain decline, based on a positive genetic test, we can refrain from judging them as immoral or unethical, although we should try to dissuade them and offer them social support. Individuals with PSEN 1 or PSEN 2 will experience a much faster progression than the usual version of Alzheimer's, which generally does not develop until someone is in their sixties or seventies and which has a slower course.

Those who test positive for PSEN 1 or PSEN 2 must ask and answer a profound question in the years before symptom onset. Some will know that they carry the mutation in their teens or twenties and know that their fate is sealed. Is Alzheimer's my destiny, in the sense of a given future that I must endure for the sake of life, God, nature, and the universe? Some will conclude, *I think not*, while others will reflect, *Well, this is the only life that I have*, or *I will trust a Higher Power*, or perhaps, *I will trust that love will find a way*.

Q: **REASON TWO:** What kind of legacy is
left behind?

A: Not a good one.

Suicide sends a message to loved ones, communities, and society that when the burdens of life are difficult to carry, suicide is an acceptable solution. It creates a legacy in the form of a family narrative. There is then a social argument against suicide. With regard to PPAS specifically, what does this practice say to the grandchildren who hear about it as they are struggling with lack of meaning and inner malaise as they try to navigate modern adolescence? Maybe PPAS imposes a burden on the young in their vulnerability and undermines the bedrock principle that we do not want to pass the torch of suicide to our children and grandchildren. This is a serious moral consideration, but not necessarily one that rises to the level that says that PPAS should be unavailable.

So many great thinkers, including Thomas Aquinas, felt that the somewhat contagious nature of suicide as an answer to life's major challenges is a primary reason not to endorse it. We are all role models. Grandma J was a great role model for self-reliance and defiance of dependence, but was she a good role model for her family? Some would say that she was courageous, independent, and even hopeful as an active agent preempting her intractable decline. Others would say that she gave up on life when the going got tough.

Q: REASON THREE: What about interdependence?

A: It needs to guide our actions.

Suicide denies the essential interdependence of human experience. Often people with a diagnosis of dementia will claim that they do not want to be burdens on family or society. But as argued in chapter one, dependence constitutes the deepest core of human experience, even when we pretend that we are in essence self-reliant. We should not deny the reality of dependence, and this fact along with the caregiving that it inevitably entails must be in the foreground of policy. In an economically just and fair society a reliable and robust support for caregivers and for deeply forgetful people is in place. Regrettably, the United States does not have much support in place, and we lag badly behind Canada and most other developed countries. Moreover, we are depriving our children of the sorts of opportunity for growth that I experienced with Grandma Post, and that helped me see that there is more "alive inside" than meets the eye, and that we are ultimately dependent beings, like it or not.

So often people who are facing a chronic illness state that they want to die because they do not want to inconvenience others, or, as one person put it, "be a leech." But how can someone be a leech if their family and devoted professionals find tremendous meaning and gratification in providing them with care? Besides, through caregiving a young person can perhaps discover the beautiful meaning of providing care—and the silver lining is that they might go on to medical school, clinical social work, nursing, or basic neuroscience. Long ago this was my silver lining when I visited Grandma Post.

Q: **REASON FOUR:** Can we learn to notice
    the expressions of selfhood?

A: Absolutely.

Another lesson that a deeply forgetful person teaches is for others to "notice" their continuing self-identity. As I have argued throughout this book, there is still the treasure of a person in the earthen vessel of an atrophied brain. Caregivers are adept at noticing the details of continuity, and they find meaning in being open to surprises that reveal this continuity. If I thought that a deeply forgetful person was ever really gone and dead in all but body, perhaps I would think that PPAS really is in the interests of someone with a probable diagnosis. But this view denies the reality of selfhood that is so widely evident to caregivers. Deep forgetfulness does not involve the loss of consciousness that we associate with the persistent vegetative state of brain death.

Q: **REASON FIVE**: Isn't hospice good enough?

A: One would hope so.

My position in chapter three seems an adequate alternative to PPAS: the refusal or cessation of any and all medical treatments for any medical need whatsoever (other than relief of pain) is ethically and legally legitimate, and this purely palliative model is the proper response to moderate and advanced Alzheimer's. This model need not be imposed on those who object to it, but it needs to be more or less standard in recommendations to families and in health care systems. Far too many deeply forgetful people are badly overtreated with tubes in every orifice, filling intensive care units and leaving medical students wondering why this practice goes on.

Why Not Legalize PPAS in the United States?

PPAS for a condition such as cancer is legal in various states but is restricted to individuals who are lucid of mind and able to make an autonomous choice, and who are also within about six months of death. (Predicting the timing of death is of course a very inexact science, so two physicians independently give their best guess.) Thus, PPAS works for people with pancreatic and other terminal cancers, and it works for patients in the end stages of ALS (amyotrophic lateral sclerosis, better known as Lou Gehrig's disease), where they are still lucid of mind and will clearly die within months due to an inability to breathe. But Alzheimer's lies outside of these laws because an individual will have lost the ability to act in their own assisted suicide at least several years before they are likely to die. Yet if PPAS is strongly desired, it is hard to justify denying deeply forgetful people the freedom to make this choice while they are able. To restate, the legal requirements for PPAS in the United States preclude dementia patients because by the time they are diagnosed with dementia, their cognitive impairments have already rendered them incapable of making a competent and informed choice (Dresser 2017). Perhaps the laws should be revised to fit those with early Alzheimer's. A diagnosis of probable Alzheimer's is a serious matter, and even those of us who advocate for deeply forgetful people against the exclusionary tendencies of a hypercognitive culture have to take their wishes seriously and be present in quiet acknowledgment of their integrity, for we cannot assert that they are acting unethically.

Caregivers need to know that PPAS is not legal in the United States at this time, even where assisted suicide laws are in place and effective for those with conditions such as terminal cancer or end-stage ALS. For better or worse, our laws in the United States, in contrast to the Netherlands, were designed mostly for people within months of death who still have cognitive as well as physical capacities to choose suicide and carry it out. One can reasonably ask if states that allow PPAS should expand their current laws to include PPAS for individuals for whom death is not immediately imminent but whose capacity for choice will soon deteriorate. However, I would not at this juncture recommend such an expansion of the law, primarily because in our nation, with such limited support for long-term care and for caregivers, I fear that PPAS would become expected due to its obvious affordability. The Dutch justify PPAS as an alternative to "self-effacement," and the ancient Stoic philosophers like Seneca justified suicide in old age when significant declines appeared imminent. Perhaps some will oppose PPAS because they do not consider Alzheimer's to be a terminal condition, although in the broadest sense it certainly is terminal and should be considered as such. While it is not imminently terminal, it is eventually so, and for those who see the inevitable decline in mental activity in the bleakest terms, it is sadly deemed terminal metaphorically—that is, in a cognitive sense (de Beaufort and de Vathorst 2016).

> Q: **CAUTION ONE:** Will PPAS diminish social commitment to long-term care?
>
> A: Quite possibly (the incompatibility hypothesis).

Even if popular referenda for PPAS are eventually passed in some states or even nationwide, the practice should ideally not be implemented until after hospice and long-term care systems for people with dementia are developed. Without the full development of affordable long-term care systems in the United States, assisted suicide would become a choice that people diagnosed with dementia might feel compelled to make, rather than one they could accept or reject. I propose to identify this concern, which has been an undercurrent in recent discussions, as the "incompatibility hypothesis"; that is, in a health care system that currently fails to provide adequate comfort care for the dying or long-term care for the dependent, legalization of PPAS for Alzheimer's disease may prove incompatible with the development of such care—and in fact is more likely to discourage it. I offer this hypothesis as a note of caution, not a full-fledged argument.

It can be argued that the concept of incompatibility is not applicable to health care. For example, acceptance of the right to withdraw or withhold life-sustaining therapy did not preclude the development of new forms of such therapy; indeed, these technologies continue to develop at a fast pace and resources are invested in them. Therefore, the argument runs, it is unlikely that the legalization of PPAS will hamper the development of other good options. Perhaps the availability of PPAS would even spur opponents of these practices to mobilize resources and develop state-of-the-art hospice and long-term care systems for deeply forgetful people. It is hard to say, but I err here on the side of caution and hope for better care systems.

Q: CAUTION TWO: Will PPAS spill over into other "nonterminal" illness categories?

A: Most likely.

This is a serious question, because Alzheimer's itself is only terminal in the broadest possible sense. A person diagnosed with Alzheimer's who does not choose PPAS might not die for many years, so critics can argue that if we define "terminal" so broadly, life itself becomes a "terminal condition"—which of course it is, unless we see break-throughs in antiaging science. So, yes, PPAS probably would spill over into "nonterminal" illness categories, which is a major problem. After all, Derek Humphry, founder of the Hemlock Society, in his controversial book *Final Exit* (1991), proposes that society accept assisted suicide and euthanasia, not just for the terminally ill but also for (a) the spouse whose loved one is dying and wishes to "go together"; (b) those with spinal cord injuries; and (c) those who are just getting old. While I disagree with Humphry, I appreciate his honesty in acknowledging that it is difficult to limit assisted suicide to the context of terminal illness. The spillover of this practice from terminal care to PPAS and then to other forms of human illness that challenge the will to live is unavoidable.

Since national guidelines were established in 1984, the Netherlands has permitted de facto assisted suicide and euthanasia, although the practice is limited to terminally ill persons, including persons with progressive dementias. Since December 1993, physicians who participate in assisted suicide and euthanasia have been excluded by law from criminal prosecution, and it has been specified that the patient must be suffering unbearably, must be in the terminal phase of illness, and must have more than once expressed the will to die. In June 1994 the Dutch Supreme Court went further. It ruled that Dr. Boudewijn Chabot could not be prosecuted for assisting in the suicide of a fifty-year-old woman who was suffering after the deaths of her two sons. Chabot's patient could not cope with life, and he decided, after seeing her for twenty-four hours in total, that her wish to die was genuine. Subsequently, "he provided her with the lethal preparation, which she drank in his presence and that of a friend and her general practitioner. Chabot then reported the case to judicial authorities as required by law" (Spanjer 1994, 1630). The Supreme Court judgment clarified that mental suffering is a legally acceptable reason for assisted suicide.

If assisted suicide is an acceptable response to mental suffering (that is applicable to people who are competent), then it is a viable option for most of us at one point or another, since few people get through life without considerable grief. Instead of pursuing psychiatric treatment through grief analysis, a rare but acceptable alternative in the Netherlands is to remove the griever himself or herself, and thereby also the grief. From this perspective, the problems of an existential nature that challenge the character of every man and woman alive no longer need to be resolved creatively; they can instead be sufficient grounds for a "final exit."

To condone by law and policy the removal of the sufferer, such as the woman in the Netherlands, is to sanction actions that cannot be narrowly contained and circumscribed. When we do so we encourage a culture in which courage, endurance, hope, love, and creativity in the face of life's burdens can be set aside and replaced by feeble purpose, low ideals, fear of discomfort, and the inability to endure disappointment without losing heart. Classically, the major arguments against suicide have been that (1) it is a usurpation of the authority of God, who both gives life and takes it away; (2) it shows a lack of faith in creative approaches to resolving relational and other difficulties; (3) it has the ripple effect of encouraging others to follow suit; and (4) it is contrary to true human nature and therefore can never be something we authentically desire. It is easy to formulate objections to both the first and fourth of these arguments. Appealing to a divine command does not carry much rational weight, and people who wish to die are not always irrational and acting in violation of human nature. The second and third, however, have some merit, especially in a time of social anomie and loss of meaning.

Who is granted permission for assisted suicide, and why, is difficult to control. My misgivings go even further, based on what the sociologist Émile Durkheim described as obligatory altruistic suicide in his classic 1897 study *Suicide* (Durkheim 1952; Berrios and Mohanna 1990). Such suicide is obligatory not by law but due to cultural expectations, as living itself comes to be viewed as selfish. Instead of being regarded as wrong or at best morally ambiguous, from this perspective suicide would come to be seen as an act of justice intended to remove undue burdens on families and society. What would initially be a choice made by the few would become an obligation for the many. The counterargument is that appeals to a hypothetical public good must be made with great care and circumspection (that is, just because assisted suicide and euthanasia are available does not mean that everyone will feel obliged to request them) (Helme 1993).

Suicide spreads. For example, Humphry's *Final Exit* describes the case of the perfectly healthy fifty-five-year-old wife of seventy-seven-year-old novelist Arthur Koestler, who drank poison with her

terminally ill husband. Yet gerontologist Robert Kastenbaum summa-
rizes a series of empirical studies indicating that suicide is not a dominant theme among elderly men and women experiencing terminal
illness. Those who survive the challenges of life and reach old age are
a tough lot with "relatively low orientation toward self-destruction."
Anger, despair, and suicidal thoughts arise "from painful conditions of life rather than from the prospect of death" (Kastenbaum
1992, 12).

Q: **CAUTION THREE:** Is there a risk of going
    from voluntary to nonvoluntary PPAS and
    even euthanasia?

A: Yes, always.

Let us clarify our terms: treatment refusal and withdrawal are common and acceptable both legally and ethically, and most patients
in hospitals die after treatments found burdensome and ineffective
have been tried and removed. PPAS, in contrast, entails the individual while still competent drinking a toxic potion by choice. Voluntary euthanasia presents an even greater contrast to PPAS: euthanasia only occurs when an individual with Alzheimer's can no longer
manage such an action but had clearly planned and intended it. In a
case of voluntary euthanasia, someone else might perform the final
act for the individual, sometimes with an advance directive for euthanasia, as allowed in the Netherlands. There is, of course, also nonvol-
untary euthanasia, which occurs when someone kills a patient even
though the patient has never indicated that they prefer to die. The
progression from PPAS to voluntary Alzheimer's euthanasia seems
to be what occurred in the Netherlands and would be a quite likely
evolution in terms of these practices—however covertly it develops.

Conclusions

The Alzheimer's Association has not taken a position for or against PPAS, which makes sense because its constituency is so divided; it is not always advisable to take positions on such a divisive issue. Having made many cautionary notes part of the discussion, we need to ask: Are they enough to outweigh a careful, informed decision to pursue PPAS? If someone with a probable diagnosis of Alzheimer's or a clearly predictive genetic test really feels that PPAS is their path, they are acting on personal conscience and do not need encouragement. I would prefer that physicians have almost nothing to do with PPAS activities because the healing arts should not mistake themselves for the suicidal or killing arts. They can work much harder to be sure that deeply forgetful people are not overtreated and that they and their families accept hospice.

Some people and their families will find hope in PPAS. Anyone who thinks that a decision to pursue PPAS is a sign of hopelessness is wrong. It can be rooted in despair, but it can also be an expression of active agency and active hope when confronted with a disease that knows no cure, delay, or prevention. Thus, I will not condemn the actions of someone like Janet Adkins as an act of despair. She saw PPAS as a path to a brighter future.

The role of health care professionals, clergy, ethicists, friends, and family of the person diagnosed with Alzheimer's who remains aware of their situation is to encourage hope in ways other than PPAS:

- Assure the person that any medical intervention in the advanced stage of Alzheimer's will only be focused on maintaining their freedom from pain and discomfort. There need be no use of artificial nutrition and hydration, no overly aggressive efforts to assist swallowing, and little recourse to antibiotics unless for palliative reasons. In essence, adhering

to a purely hospice approach to care is to be assured in advanced illness and even earlier.

· Assure the person that, while this is a disease that affects
  cognition, function, and behavior, some of its symptoms can
  be mitigated through relational, social, musical, and creative
  arts programs that can enhance their quality of life even in
  the advanced stages of the disease.

· Assure the person that dependence on others is a natural
  and inevitable aspect of human life and love, and that he or
  she can entrust himself or herself to those caring others.

At least by giving people with dementia hope for dignified, state-
funded long-term care, we make the appeal of PPAS less powerful,
although for some, the very idea of enduring this loss of memory and
cognition will remain unthinkable. *Most people with a diagnosis of Alzheimer's, if they know that they will receive the care and respect of others and
that they will not be held hostage to our technological-mechanical epoch of
protracted morbidity, would prefer to die a natural death in the midst of loved
ones.* There is enough hope for most people with dementia in the cultivation of an ethos of solicitous care and enhanced quality of life
rather than in suicide, but this is not true for all. In the end, "Judge
not lest ye be judged" (Matthew 7:1).

5

A Caregiver's Ethical Purpose

Preserving Dignity, Ten Manifestations of Care, and Respect for the Whole Story of a Life

N*ever think that an individual who is cognitively intact and has a sharp memory is of any greater moral worth than a person who is deeply forgetful.* Perhaps the most important moral opportunity we have is to affirm the dignity of deeply forgetful people through compassionate action and non-harm.

Dignity

What is dignity? Most would define it as "the quality of being worthy of honor and respect."

My interactions with deeply forgetful people affirm that the basis for living human dignity is consciousness itself and nothing more. The basis is not in reasoning, however refined, limited, or even non-existent. Philosophers as far back as the ancient Stoics and even Plato have often named rationality as the one property that affords moral status, and they generally define rationality procedurally—as an ability to do certain things, such as to act consistently based on clear thinking, to arrive at decisions by deliberation, to envisage a future for oneself, and so forth. But in fact very few of us live our lives in a consistently rational way (Zagzebski 2001), and many people make a habit of meditating in order to slow their minds down and empty themselves of thoughts.

While I do not place any moral weight on rationality as the capacity to make decisions, I do recognize rationality as a source of self-identity—of who we are rather than of how we proceed to act in the world. The human mind responds to all kinds of symbols in its environment. We live in symbols and symbols live in us. I have known many deeply forgetful people who could not engage in conversation or reasoning but would smile broadly when they saw a picture of their old home or held a sacred object like a rosary in their hands. This is what I mean by the rationality of who we are rather than of how we proceed. None of these individuals had procedural reasoning skills, but they knew who they were in relation to familiar objects, voices, and attachments. While it is true that even in the more advanced stages of dementia the symbolic self will usually persist, this is perhaps not always the case, and therefore it is not the basis for unconditional dignity.

What clearly persists is consciousness, so that has to be the basis of unconditional dignity and respect.

Second, there is the conditional dignity we possess based on our character, the virtues we manifest, the kindness in our hearts, our persistence in noble causes and purposes, our dreams and ideals, our loyalty to others, our self-care, and so much else. Thus, we hear it said, "Oh, she has such a special dignity in how she responds to the challenges of life."

In many of the vignettes presented in this book caregivers state that despite a loved one's loss of health and memory his graceful manners and gentleness were preserved. It goes without saying that this is not always the case, for very dignified people can spiral down into aggressive and difficult behaviors, or even become shockingly disinhibited.

It is a caregiver's conviction that of course unconditional dignity is always there in a loved one regardless of cognitive state or diminished memory. But caregivers also affirm conditional dignity and make every effort to notice its expression even if it seems at times to grow faint. They are at work every day preserving dignity.

Four Stories of Enduring Dignity

Let me give some examples of this conditional dignity in deeply forgetful people as I have encountered them.

Jim's Glorious Twig

I met Jim, a man with advanced dementia, in a nursing home in Chardon, Ohio. I had read the sketch about Jim on the door of his room. Dr. Joe Foley and I asked the nurse on the special care unit to point him out to me. I approached, calling Jim calmly by name as if to get an answer even if one did not come. I guided Jim to a table and we sat down. I asked him how his sons were, first Jim Jr. and then Ned. He could not respond, although I have no idea what he may have understood. Then he handed me a lovely white painted twig about two feet long, which I accepted with a smile and a "Thanks, Jim." Then he smiled, and responded with three words, "God is love." If joy were electric the place would have been in flames. He was radiant, purely radiant. I was in awe of Jim. I handed the twig back to him, and he continued to smile. Dr. Foley observed all of this with a quiet affirming presence. Later, the nurse told me that when Jim was a boy, his father had given him the daily chore of bringing kindling in for the fireplace. Now, he was reliving that boyhood by doing something he associated with fatherly love and also with his Methodist theological background.

How dignified his action was! Of course, Jim had the same unconditional human dignity that we all have simply by being a living human being, but he also maintained a quality of kindness and even of intense joy in our mostly nonverbal interaction that has stayed with me for decades. As I drove back from Chardon to Cleveland with my mentor, Dr. Foley, we devoted a full hour of conversation to the subtle qualities of dignity that Jim possessed. Of course, my interaction with Jim may have been particularly revealing of this conditional dignity because he expressed his continuing character in an especially vivid action. But I was able to notice it and respond, eliciting his surprising three-word statement. Jim had plenty of dignity, both unconditional and conditional, and he exhibited a joyful grace that I would not expect to find in very many everyday encounters.

Jan's Awesome New Snowflakes

People with dementia continue to seek meaning, experience awe, and know love. The following story—only lightly edited—was told by a woman in her forties with relatively early-onset dementia whose cause was unknown. I knew Jan and her husband in Shaker Heights, Ohio, and was aware that she was an excellent writer. I asked her, with her husband's support, if she could sketch out her experiences in a brief reflection. Here is what she wrote and then read at a support group meeting of the local Alzheimer's chapter:

> It was just about this time three years ago that I recall laughing with my sister while in dance class at my turning the big four-oh. "Don't worry, life begins at forty," she exclaimed, and then

sweetly advised her younger sister of all the wonders in life still to be found. Little did either of us realize what a cruel twist life was proceeding to take. It was a fate neither she nor I ever imagined someone in our age group could encounter.

Things began to happen that I just couldn't understand. There were times I addressed friends by the wrong name. Comprehending conversations seemed almost impossible. My attention span became quite short. Notes were needed to remind me of things to be done and how to do them. I would slur my speech, use inappropriate words, or simply eliminate one from a sentence. This caused me not only frustration but also a great deal of embarrassment. Then came the times I honestly could not remember how to plan a meal or shop for groceries.

One day, while out for a walk on my usual path in a city in which I had resided for eleven years, nothing looked familiar. It was as if I was lost in a foreign land, yet I had the sense to ask for directions home.

There were more days than not when I was perfectly fine; but to me, they did not make up for the ones that weren't. I knew there was something terribly wrong, and after eighteen months of undergoing a tremendous amount of tests and countless visits to various doctors, I was proven right.

Dementia is the disease, they say, cause unknown. At this point it no longer mattered to me just what that cause was because the tests eliminated the reversible ones, my hospital coverage was gone, and my spirit was too worn to even care about the name of something irreversible.

I was angry. I was broken and this was something I could not fix, nor to date can anyone fix it for me. How was I to live without myself? I wanted her back!

She was a strong and independent woman. She always tried so hard to be a loving wife, a good mother, a caring friend, and a dedicated employee. She had self-confidence and enjoyed life. She never imagined that by the age of 41 she would be forced into retirement. She had not yet observed even one of her sons graduate from college, or known the pleasures of a daughter-in-law, or held a grandchild in her arms.

Needless to say, the future did not look bright. The leader must now learn to follow. Adversities in life were once looked upon as a challenge; now they're just confusing situations that someone else must handle. Control of my life will slowly be relinquished to others. I must learn to trust—completely.

An intense fear enveloped my entire being as I mourned the loss of what was and the hopes and dreams that might never be. How could this be happening to me? What exactly will become of me? These questions occupied much of my time for far too many days.

Then one day as I fumbled around the kitchen to prepare a pot of coffee, something caught my eye through the window. It had snowed and I had truly forgotten what a beautiful sight a soft, gentle snowfall could be. I eagerly but slowly dressed and went outside to join my son, who was shoveling our driveway. As I bent down to gather a mass of those radiantly white flakes on my shovel, it seemed as though I could do nothing but marvel at their beauty. Needless to say, my son did not share in my enthusiasm; to him it was a job, but to me it was an experience.

Later I realized that for a short period of time, God granted me the ability to see a snowfall through the innocent eyes of the child I once was, many years ago. I am still here, I thought, and there will be wonders to behold in each new day; they are just different now.

Quality of life is different to me now from the way it was before. I am very loved, in the early stages, and now my husband and my sons give back in love what I gave them. I am blessed because I am loved. That woman who killed herself—you know, with that suicide doctor—she didn't have to wind up that way. Not that I condemn her, but our lives can't really be that bad. Her choice is understandable if she wasn't loved or cared for. Now my quality of life is feeding the dogs, looking at flowers. My husband says I am more content now than ever before! Love and dignity, those are the keys. This brings you back down to the basics in life, a smile makes you happy.

This reflection is quite profound. Jan is referring in the last paragraph to Janet Adkins, who followed the path of PPAS that was discussed in chapter four. Her recognition that love gives her the strength and will to continue on into the uncharted future is powerful, for otherwise she might have wanted to enlist the same sort of assistance. But what really comes through is her deep feeling of awe before the newly fallen snow, which seemed to have an almost childlike quality of pure freshness. Her dignity was in her purity, her love of nature, and her appreciation for those who cared for her.

Ruth's Deep Gratitude

Here is Leo's story of his sense of his wife Ruth's dignity as she was recently given a probable diagnosis of Alzheimer's:

> My wife, Ruth, was told she had probable Alzheimer's. She appreciated this because it gave her something to hang her hat on. She could tell people that she was ill and that she couldn't help her forgetfulness. We accelerated plans for travel, traveling all around the United States. Ruth especially loved the fall colors in New England and the ranches in Texas. In the nursing home, we still traveled in a way by walking around the wooded paths surrounding the home. Ruth used to whistle at birds and I sometimes felt that they understood her. She would gaze at a colorful flower for ten or fifteen minutes, all the time with a smile. Sometimes, with fractured words and sentences, she would say, "I love you." She still recognizes me, but not our thirty-year-old daughter, although she has glimmers of recognition of her. Ruth spontaneously whistles and she is able to keep time with music. She likes only soft music now. When she is agitated, music can help. She still smiles a lot. A touch on the arm from a friendly person

is always well received. The key is what the person with dementia feels goes into creating a good quality of life, and we have to
work at that level. Her response to music is declining now. How
much should we try to restore her health? I oppose feeding tubes.
As Ruth declines more, I want to withhold feeding. She will have
to be moved to another nursing home that allows this. The goal
is comfort, not life prolongation. She still knows who I am, she
feels me, and she still loves me.

Leo sees so many things in Ruth, but notices in particular her whis-
tling and her smiling. Here he cares to notice Ruth's continuing qualities of lightheartedness and serenity that are still apparent. It is also
worth noting that he could see dignity in allowing her an eventual
natural death devoid of the feeding tubes that are both annoying to
the patient and by no means preferable to assisted oral feeding so
long as it is possible to do so.

Clint's Cowboy Hat

Sharen Eckert, a former director of Alzheimer's Cleveland (who herself eventually died of Alzheimer's), told me the story of her father,
who held on to his dignity until the very end, she said. He wore his
favorite cowboy hat in the shower, slept with it on his head, and
never let it out of his sight, even after entering the nursing home.
Somehow he knew that there was something special about this hat,
that it was somehow connected with who he was. While he could no
longer talk much, and never coherently, he could still play a pretty
good game of pinochle long after he forgot Sharen's name.

"He never read books much anyway," remarked Sharen. "He
worked in the steel mills and had lots of male drinking friends. People of intellectual capabilities would not have appreciated Dad's many
moments of joy. Of course, there were down moments for Dad too,

like there are for everyone. But his quality of life cannot be adequately evaluated by the intellectuals, who are not a jury of his peers."

Clint knew that he was that country-and-western-style worker from the steel mills on Cleveland's west side, and that he had worked hard and lived a good life in the culture of that world. He was preserving his dignity by staying close to his hat, which, according to "object relations" theory, reminded him of who he was.

Acting against Indignity and Humiliation

An essential task of any caregiver is to advocate for deeply forgetful people whenever and wherever possible so as to defend their unconditional and conditional dignity.

The Nazi Doctors and the Perils of Forgetfulness

All good health care professionals affirm the dignity of deeply forgetful people. It is a test of their character and depth. But this was not so a century ago in Germany. The Nazi doctors, with their rigid association of cognitive strength and moral status despite the Hippocratic oath to "do no harm," subjected deeply forgetful people as "life unworthy of life" to horrific hypothermia experiments. The doctors who conducted these experiments were steeped in eugenic ideas about human progress—ideas rooted in the thought of Francis Galton—about how the few who are more intelligent than most should propagate their superior genes. The "imbeciles" and the deeply forgetful could rightly be eliminated.

We see nothing so extreme being attempted today in part because advocacy organizations are so effective, based on the arguments of Dr. Leo Alexander, the primary author of the famous Nuremberg

Code of 1947 (Alexander 1949). Indeed, in my view the main role of an advocacy organization like the Alzheimer's Association is to advocate socially and politically for the dignity and moral standing of deeply forgetful people, as well as for psychosocial interventions that work wonders.

Outright cruelty is clearly visible in early hypothermia experiments like T-4, in 1939, when thirty thousand persons with dementia were taken from German mental asylums and left outdoors overnight to freeze in the cold winter air (Muller-Hill 1988). Because memory is a form of power, we can sometimes find in those who have lost such power the opportunity to mock or ignore, sending the message that their very existence rests on a mistake (Post 2000).

More generally, because we fear loss of cognitive strength, we sadly tend to demean those whose capacity to remember has dissipated by treating them with indifference or even cruelty. This indifference is obvious when we approach a person with dementia and neglect to speak with them directly, or to make eye contact with them, or to call them by their name and expect a response. It could be the waiter in a restaurant or the doctor in the clinic, but there is a tendency to talk around or about someone with dementia, rather than with them.

Here are two powerful situations in which I have stepped into the struggle against de-dignification.

The Stark Humiliation of Mrs. H

In the summer of 2004 I was asked to provide a court deposition on behalf of the Muslim son of a woman who had been raped in a nursing home. Mrs. H had been faithfully married for many years before her husband died. Following the dictates of Islam and of her local imam, Mrs. H had neither dated nor been sexually intimate for ten years after her spouse's passing. Then came her diagnosis of probable Alzheimer's disease and her eventual placement in a nursing home. Mrs. H was a wanderer, and one night she ambled down the hall into the bedroom of a somewhat younger resident with mild learning difficulties and a history of sexual aggression. An evening nurse, who made fifteen-minute checks on Mrs. H, discovered the two naked and in the bed. Mrs. H was weeping. Several days later, Mrs. H was able to mention this incident to her Muslim daughter-in-law, but she was fearful of bringing it directly to the attention of her son, who also practiced Islam, for there was family dishonor associated with being raped. The son brought a legal suit against the nursing home for negligence, and I was asked to give a deposition.

The attorney defending the nursing home argued that, in fact, even though Mrs. H was apparently briefly upset about the violation of her long-established religious values and about this assault itself, she soon forgot about the incident. Therefore, the defense attorney argued, she had not experienced significant "lasting" harm, and thus the case was frivolous—if indeed she did actually express her grief and agitation to her daughter-in-law over having been sexually intimate, and if indeed she really could have authentic religious commitments at her stage of dementia.

In a three-hour-long deposition, I argued that significant harm was done. First, Mrs. H was harmed with respect to her remaining self-identity, for she was a deeply committed Muslim throughout her life and still found meaning in her faith as evidenced by occasional moments of prayer and a protective attitude toward sacred objects in her room. While she had lost a significant portion of her memory, there were episodes of insight into her past and her belief system. Thus, it was wrong to assert that the sporadic nature of her insights made the violation of her self-identity unimportant. Instead of dismissing her past as irrelevant, I suggested, we should work to create an environment in which her connections with the past are cultivated in order to enhance her sense of security and well-being. Second, Mrs. H was harmed emotionally even if she recovered from her agitation quickly, because she could not retain vivid memories of what had occurred after several days had passed. The emotional life of Mrs. H is an aspect of her experience that should be especially respected as the source of her well-being and quality of life. Yet at every turn, the defending lawyer mounted intense counterarguments, most of which amounted to the assertion that someone who is demented cannot experience harm with regard to self-identity or affect, at least not in any significant "lasting" manner. And in response, I continued to assert that the cognitive, autobiographical, emotional, relational, and sentient aspects of the deeply forgetful should be respected, just as they are in humans whose memories have not yet faded much. (For readers who are curious, I should add that the case was settled out of court—in favor of Mrs. H.)

Dignity in the Parking Lot

One day I was standing in the parking lot in front of a clinic, and I witnessed a difficult late afternoon scene. An elderly woman in the passenger seat of a car was being yelled at by her husband, who was in the driver's seat. It was a warm day and the windows were open. I heard this: "What the hell, you can't even figure out how to open the door! You [chain of expletives] useless pointless pile of garbage! I wish I had never married you, and look at you now. You can't even open the damned door, you fool!" Then he slammed his fist into the ceiling of the car as his wife whimpered and shook in fear. She began to cry deeply.

I walked over to the car and knocked gently on the husband's door. "Hey, sir, let's just walk around the car and open her door for her. I can help you."

He was a little embarrassed, and together we walked his wife into the clinic. As they sat down I told him that I knew he was having a hard time, but that we could connect him with a really good clinical social worker who could improve things a bit, and that he and his wife should come to an Alzheimer's Association support group that evening in the same building, which they did. I saw them there and we had some time for a positive conversation.

With Association support and coaching, this husband turned out to be a good caregiver. He confided that his wife had been very good to him over the years, and that now was his chance to be good to her. Over time, we became friends.

The Circle of Care: Ten Manifestations

Caregivers perform their amazing daily feats because they affirm the dignity of deeply forgetful people. They see their worth, both unconditional and conditional. *Because they see the dignity, they can sustain the love.* In this section, I will use "care" and "love" synonymously.

The psychiatrist Harry Stack Sullivan of the University of Chicago wrote, "When the happiness, security, and well-being of another person is as real to you, or more real, than your own, you love that person." We can all relate to this definition of love, whether we are contemplating friendship, parenthood, a special calling to assist a needy group, or affirming our shared humanity. The centrality of such love in the everyday lives of caregivers should be obvious. Care is an expression of their love.

This loving care has many modulations, depending on the needs of deeply forgetful people. Each "way of love" constitutes a spoke on the wheel in the figure, and caregivers engage in all these expressions of care and surely others that are not listed here.

- Celebration is taking time to acknowledge and affirm the lives and achievements of others.
- Helping others in ways small and large without being limited by a "payback" mentality is as good for the giver as for the recipient.
- Forgiveness is breaking free from destructive emotions by concentrating not on our own resentments but on contributing to the lives of others and knowing that time will put things in deeper perspective.

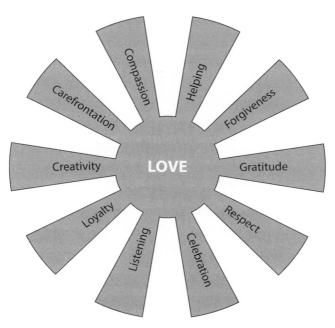

Ten ways of caring for deeply forgetful people.

- Carefrontation is standing firm against the destructive behavior of individuals and society, while staying grounded in an underlying love for all people without exception.
- Mirth is the gift of tastefully reframing a situation with loving laughter that does not diminish but rather uplifts; mirth is the lightness of love.
- Respect (*respectare*, or "re-look") means looking more carefully at the opinions and lives of others, striving for civility in discourse, and practicing etiquette in speech and behavior.
- Attentive listening is setting aside one's own voice in order to focus on another with a full presence, undistracted and unhurried.
- Compassion is responding wisely and actively to suffering when we see it.
- Loyalty is sticking with others through the peaks and valleys of their lives so they know that they can count on you in tough times.
- Creativity used for noble purposes is the tool that allows unique, personalized expression of our love for others.

The Way of Celebration

Love means rejoicing in the presence of another, in that person's simply being alive, and in his or her achievements. Rejoicing holds a central role in most spiritual traditions: "O give thanks unto the Lord, for he is good: for his mercy endureth for ever" (Psalms 107:1).

Rejoice in the newness of life each day. Be open to surprises. Rejoice together with your loved one in the red and gold of autumn leaves; for cloud and sun, hills and streams, ice and snow; for trees in spring, and fruit blossoms, and birds; for the smell of the earth after rain; for fireside and friendly conversation; for meals eaten together in fellowship; for games; for walks; for times in the open air; for birthdays, festivals, and holidays; for musicians and painters, poets and artisans. Yes, it is possible to celebrate with a deeply forgetful person. Imagine how loveless life would be without rejoicing and celebration.

The Way of Helping

If your loved one is up to it, ask them to help you with some tangible deed to improve the community. Suffering and compassion need not be involved. Be a helper, be a neighbor. Rake the leaves, take out the garbage, shovel a little snow. Do some volunteering together. The helping that goes on in everyday life, in the home, between friends, at work or school, or with a stranger at the food line, allows a deeply forgetful person to feel gratified. This kind of behavior occurs in the wonderful intergenerational schools across the country when the deeply forgetful renew their bright smile and even regain some inspiration when trying to help a youngster read a children's book. I knew a man in Shaker Heights, Ohio, who was diagnosed with Alzheimer's and became quite rapidly forgetful. But, lo and behold, he loved to ride in the passenger seat of the van that would pick people up to attend the Alzheimer's art session, and he would help them walk from the door of their home to the van, and then into the Foley Elder Healthcare Center. He received so much from discovering this source of happiness, and he continued on for two years!

Sometimes when I was bored as a child, my mom would say, "Stevie, why don't you just go out and help someone?" And I would go across the street and give old Mr. Muller a hand raking leaves. It always felt pretty good. Again, there wasn't anything especially deep and profound about it. These are just activities that connect us together in a web of helpfulness.

The Way of Forgiveness

Forgiving is a big part of caregiving. A loved one will do all kinds of things that are aggravating and tend to cause us to react. It is so easy for a caregiver to lose patience, to snap, to lose inner control in re-sponse to a deeply forgetful person. The way of forgiveness requires a lot of inner discipline so as not to react but rather to respond with kindness. For a caregiver, every day managing diapers requires some sort of forgiveness.

The Way of Carefrontation

Sometimes a caregiver has to try to get through to a loved one and see if they can correct a difficult behavior. "Carefrontation" means confronting people with destructive or self-destructive behaviors and attitudes in a quite compassionate way that allows them to still feel cared for, significant, and hopeful for change. It is about giving criti-cal feedback without humiliation.

The Way of Mirth

I have known some deeply forgetful people who could really appreci-ate a simple joke. Never rebuke the merry. I once knew a wonderful preacher who carried two books everywhere: the Gospels and a col-lection of tasteful jokes for all occasions. There is much good achieved in cheering up the world. Some of us are called by our nature to be love's jesters. The great entertainer Bob Hope lived to the age of one hundred. What made him so great? Over seven decades, his mirth and laughter brought smiles to millions, and a healthy tasteful humor cultivated hope in troops stationed in war zones across the world. He would always have time for a quiet moment with a wounded soldier, no matter how tired he might be from a long flight or a busy schedule. Bob Hope spent a lot of time in nursing homes and in special care units with deeply forgetful people. His mirthfulness, his natural joy, carried over to them. And often after singing a song that they could easily recall from their generational cohort, he could share a few jokes and people across the room would all smile and laugh.

It is always good for a caregiver to find some way to smile and laugh at times. Love can be expressed in levity, and angels fly because of their lightness. It is hard to imagine loving someone you can't laugh with, at least a little. Laughter frees us from anxiety or despair. When we laugh, the ego self seems to disappear. Our worries just go out the window. We forget about the weight of life and experience a new beginning. Humor distracts us from the constant march and demands of chronological time.

I have seen caregivers use a lot of laughter in communicating with a loved one. This is sporadic and not always possible, of course, but never think that a deeply forgetful person cannot enjoy an episode of *The Three Stooges* or *The Little Rascals*. As a caregiver, laugh at your mistakes and embrace your imperfection. Perfection can be the enemy of laughter. Proverbs 17:22 reads, "A cheerful heart is a good medicine."

True, caregiving is no joyride. But the fact that there is suffering in our lives and in the lives of others is no excuse for the repression of mirth.

The Way of Respect

Respect touches on a sort of emotional awe or reverence. By this I mean an emotional sense of quiet amazement over the existence of another person, a sense of miracle and wonder over his or her unique qualities, a basic acceptance of that person without seeking to refashion the beloved into a replica of oneself. Minimally, this implies an unwillingness to overpower or manipulate, and an appreciation for the freedom of the beloved as he or she navigates the journey of life. Respect does not seek to absorb the other into the self, but recognizes and accepts the other as other, while retaining an intense interest. Respect, as an affective expression of love, is the calm awe that underlies an abiding humility. In this sense, love keeps its distance even as it draws near, and contains a certain hesitation as it holds the other inviolable.

Respect demands that we look twice and three times at others, seeking to understand their personal histories, their struggles, their life journeys. A great deal of human cruelty stems directly from an irreverent unwillingness to respect the thoughts, feelings, and lives of others.

This entire book has been a statement of the immense respect that caregivers often have for their loved ones.

The Way of Attentive Listening

A caregiver has to be a highly sensitive listener to find the meaning that a loved one is trying to convey in words and behaviors. The caregiver is the one who listens attentively in order to understand; reassurance, consolation, comfort, and advice flow from this listening. To be human is to speak, and to be a healer is to listen. Those who work with people in crisis know that often the only thing they have to offer is an attentive listening presence. We wish that there was some medication that would help deeply forgetful people, but there is really nothing that can be done other than being present, listening, and really hearing in an affirming way. This is not so easy because we have to turn off our usual talkativeness and enter a kind of holy attentiveness to the other that is completely unconditional, meeting people where they are, as they are, and allowing them to find comfort in your simply being there.

The Way of Compassion

Deeply forgetful people do suffer in many ways at times. They can suffer early on because they are insightful about their losses and *do not yet forget that they forget.* Later on they may suffer because they are overwhelmed by the confused and confusing world coming at them. They may miss a familiar item of deep attachment, like a doll or a special hat that has great meaning to them based on their earlier lives. Compassion is the ability to feel the suffering of others to some degree, and to respond actively to reduce that suffering. The Good Samaritan (Luke 10:30–35) sees a man suffering on the roadside, and "is moved by compassion." The man had been beaten by robbers, who left him stripped and half dead. The Samaritan "had compassion," and he bound up the man's wounds, took him to an inn, and cared for him, even paying his bill. It is all so immediate and direct.

A Buddhist will contend that we may not be suffering at this very moment, but things will change in this world of *dukkha* (suffering). We may have a great job, plenty of friends, a good marriage, wonderful children, and good health. In the next moment, any or all of these things may disappear. Of course, the smiling Buddha will tell us to fully enjoy good fortune and to savor the sunny days of life, partly because suffering always lurks around the corner, even in the best of times. There is much truth to this Buddhist philosophy. Yet, the idea of this lurking suffering seems a bit overstated to me. There are times of immense joy, creative flow, and meaningful generativity that seem to entirely escape suffering, even in some nagging sense of potentiality. Still, at a deeper level, we are all broken by different things along the journey of life. We all carry wounds and regrets, some of which are of our own making and some are received from others.

This discussion brings us back again to the artist Willem de Kooning, who had a reputation for getting in a lot of drunken brawls in Greenwich Village. He seems to have suffered a lot of anxiety with life. But after he was diagnosed with dementia, he drifted away from suffering and his painting became so much more tranquil and uplifting. He came to forget that he forgot, and peace ensued. He still had difficult moments, for sure, but he loved to paint and that is what he did with help for years until he passed away.

The Way of Loyalty

Caregivers are the most loyal people on earth. They have to be. They also need to know when to bring their loved one to a nursing home because they cannot handle the complexities of care anymore. But that is still an act of loyalty so long as they visit every day or every few days and help out. A nursing home placement is not a broken covenant, just a geographical relocation. For many decades, older adults have rightly extracted a promise from their loved ones: "Please, never put me in a nursing home!" This is because the nursing home model did little more than warehouse older adults, especially those who had any degree of memory deficit, and treated them entirely in terms of a medical model that focused primarily on their physical needs. Overly objective and pacifying, this model tends to treat older adults as biological substrates rather than as human beings capable of choice, purpose, creativity, prosocial activities, and meaningful emotion and relationality. No wonder older adults have feared the nursing home. Fortunately, there has been a major grassroots effort to change from a medical to a person-centered model of care that takes older adults—including the deeply forgetful ones—seriously as active agents in daily life. Organizations such as the Pioneer Network have focused on a culture change that enhances the lives of older adults within environments that nurture their remaining capacities. So, when a caregiver places a loved one in a nursing home because things have become too difficult, this is not a betrayal anymore, because the caregiver can now partner with a team and do something wonderful.

Deeply forgetful people seek constancy in relationship and presence. You may think that they are not aware of who you are as a caregiver, but in almost all cases they maintain their attachments to loved ones and are upset by separation. Caregivers express love in fidelity and permanence over time. Constancy provides security and safety. Constancy means being committed in one's relationships. Herein is an emotional safe haven, and a security of attachment that every newborn requires, and that we never stop requiring over the course of a lifetime. And herein is the possibility for a deepening of relationship over time despite the unforeseen. In other words, growth can only unfold with constancy.

Deeply forgetful people are indeed a bit tattered of brain. But Tom Smith, the horse trainer in the movie *Seabiscuit*, looks over at a pretty tattered horse and says, "Don't ever throw away a whole life just because it's a little banged up." Loyalty requires patience and forbearance and tolerance. No relationship will last long without these elements.

Deeply forgetful people experience fallen self-esteem, bewildering isolation, anxiety, and haunting depressions. They need stable love over time, the love that serves as the glue between past, present, and future.

The Way of Creativity

Deeply forgetful people can be amazingly creative in art, music, and many other things. Caregivers need to nurture that creativity as an expression of love. Any good nursing home will have walls covered with quite wonderful paintings and watercolors done by deeply forgetful people. Allowing them to be creative means so very much to them, and it allows a caregiver to know that their loved one is still there in lots of ways. I knew a woman who had a diagnosis of Alzheimer's. "When I got home," she told me, "I would start knitting, a pastime that I had always found calming. It would not take long before I had a pretty colorful lap blanket. I made a few, and then it came to me—I could bring these to the Alzheimer's Center to brighten up the place."

Each caregiver will manifest love in many of these ten ways over the course of the day. They use their gifts to enhance quality of life for a loved one, relying on innovative vision and creativity. Caregivers are some of the most creative people on earth.

Respect for the Whole Story of a Life

Respect is a modulation of love. When we disrespect someone it means that we are not looking deeply or carefully enough to take them seriously or regard them as equals. Disrespect comes naturally to human beings because we are so caught up in seeing people around us as means to our own goals, and more generally because we view the world through the lens of our own minds and feelings simply by being separate embodied beings. We tend to be preoccupied with our own concerns and anxieties, making us inattentive, both in our seeing and in our listening. Respect is mostly in the details, in noticing

the small things that are often of large consequence, such as someone's tone of voice or facial expression.

When we respect a deeply forgetful person we are also respecting
ourselves, because forgetfulness occurs on a spectrum from mild to
severe. Again, we are all forgetful, and we are all deeply forgetful at
times, though we differ in the consistency and duration of our episodes of deep forgetfulness. We are all surprised or even worried by
our forgetfulness at times, and we wonder why our memories sporadically fail us only to return a little later. We might say something
like, "Oh, it will come back to me in a little while. Goodness, how
embarrassing." In these moments there is no doubt in our mind that
we are still "there," with our life narrative intact, despite a fleeting
memory lapse. This rather benign forgetfulness is more significant
in what is called "normal" age-related memory loss, but most people
experience it in varying degrees throughout their lives. But we begin
to worry when we begin to forget more often. Further along on this
continuum are the more deeply forgetful ones who need reminders
more than most, especially with names and words that were once on
the tip of their tongues. But once again, we do not doubt that their
self-identity is still there. A person with dementia is just further along
this spectrum to various degrees, still "there" and sometimes much
more aware of their lapses than they can express in language—hence
their frustrated and agitated behaviors. They may also forget that
they forget, which is a blessing of a sort because they then are no longer anxious about their memories.

We respect deeply forgetful people because with the right stimulation specific memories will come back to them because they were
not really gone as much as hidden away. The surprising revelations
of selfhood are a common occurrence, including well-documented
instances of terminal lucidity before dying.

The Example of Sexual Intimacy and Integrity

One way we disrespect deeply forgetful people is by separating who they are in the now from who they were in the past. The radical differentiation between the formerly intact or "then" self and the currently demented or "now" self, as advanced by some commentators, is simply a misrepresentation of the facts. The reality is that until the very advanced and even terminal stage of dementia, an individual will usually retain long-term, and sporadically articulated, memories of deeply meaningful events and relationships. It is dangerous nonsense to bifurcate, in any absolute sense, the self into "then" and "now," because doing so denigrates the integrity of the "then" self that never really exists only in the past because of the many ways in which deeply forgetful people have a continuing self-identity (Post 1995a)— continuities that are occasionally quite evident. This is why it is essential that professional caregivers be aware of the person's life story, do all they can to respect the integrity of that story, and compensate for the person's memory losses by providing cues that can help them maintain continuity in self-consciousness. Even in the advanced stage of dementia, as in Leo's story about his wife Ruth, one finds varying degrees of emotional and relational expression, remnants of personality, and even meaningful nonverbal communication, such as reaching out for a hug.

Family and professional caregivers have identified sexual ethics as a major area where guidance is needed when caring for the deeply forgetful. Once when I was working with the Eastern Massachusetts chapter of the Alzheimer's Association, the following episode was described by a professional caregiver from a local nursing home:

> In our nursing home, Mrs. J. was pretty severely demented. She was completely unable to recognize her husband. He would

come into the nursing home and insist on exercising his conjugal rights. And yes, he was totally adamant about this. So we allowed him to enter his wife's room. I can tell you that she didn't know her husband from Adam, and that she had no apparent interest in sex. After several episodes of what, from my perspective, was more or less like rape, we told the husband that he should forget about his conjugal rights, and look elsewhere for satisfaction.

There was general consensus regarding the nursing home's stated position, needless to say. In this case, the husband stopped coming by the nursing home for sex. Yet the case is a poignant one, since the couple had been married for many years, had raised children, and had been generally happy together.

I recall a woman in Boise, Idaho, who spoke up about her experiences as a family caregiver for her husband, whose dementia caused a seemingly indefatigable desire for sexual intercourse. Her husband had become both disinhibited and relatively aggressive, and his heightened desires went far beyond anything she felt physically or emotionally comfortable with. This situation was very stressful for her, because when she turned him away he became very agitated and even more aggressive, to the point where she had to place him in a nursing home. This particular caregiver was moved to tears, not just because of the unmanageable sexual desires of her husband, but because of the painful reality that, when making love to her, he seemed to have little idea of who she was and would sometimes call her by names other than her own. Similar cases are well documented through interviews with other caregiving wives in a remarkable empirical study by Linda K. Wright (1993).

While working on ethical issues with caregivers and professionals in the Toronto area, I had the good fortune of meeting Susan Hart, who provided advice to caregivers in her position with the Alzheimer Society of York Region. Hart's splendid caregiver guidebook

(*Lady from the Center*, 1997) is deeply grounded in her years of experience with this constituency. She includes a thoughtful discussion entitled "Sexual Relationships and Other Challenges." It begins with the following passage, so practical and down to earth:

> A progressive dementia is a disinhibitor. With it come behavioral changes! The fact is that these changes can be translated into increased sexual activities. Before I continue you should understand that THIS BEHAVIOR IS NOT CHARACTERISTIC OF ALL PROGRESSIVE DEMENTIA. It is, however, sufficiently common that greater discussion and understanding should take place. In the most serious cases, the individual constantly wants sexual satisfaction. This translates into groping, suggestions, anger, and accusations. The level of comprehension of the act itself and the emotions involved are not present. There is only one basic need. I have known men and women who still share the same bed and wake up several times during the night with hands exploring in a most devastating and, as they say, degrading manner. In situations such as this, guilt about not wanting to be a willing partner causes most caregivers to try to complete the sexual act only to find within a short time that interest and ability have been lost. This then can start up again within a very short time. (Hart 1997, 41)

Hart goes on to describe cases where "bending over to do care is an invitation to have a blouse undone or a zipper pulled down" (Hart 1997, 42). This is anything but welcome, Hart continues, for the caregiver who is already worn out, "and slowly but surely being smothered to death with the physical act of care giving while attempting to avoid the unusual sexual demands of a stranger," that is, a husband who seems like a stranger and may be requesting acts not part of the marriage prior to dementia and which she finds repugnant. Hart offers various practical suggestions, from twin beds to refusing such advances in a tone of voice that is firm yet kind.

Hart's presentation highlights the seriousness of the kind of dementia that causes disinhibition and hypersexuality. Should an already burdened caregiver accept demands for physical intimacy with a spouse who is in a disinhibited state of repeated sexual arousal? Despite the emotionally and physically difficult circumstances, many women caregivers try to accommodate such demands, but they also learn to draw boundaries. The best solution for both the informal family caregiver and the loved one is indeed often the nursing home. No caregiver should feel guilty about this decision. In many cases, there comes a time when it is unavoidable.

The nursing home situation can itself be emotionally complex for the caregiver, however, who on visits may see a life partner behaving like an uninhibited romantic adolescent. In one case a woman with advanced Alzheimer's was hallucinating and projecting the presence of her long-deceased husband onto another man in the special care unit. That man was still somewhat intact mentally and responded to her expressions of affection as though they were an invitation to his last sexual tango. On one of his better days, the man requested cohabitation privileges. The nursing staff approached the woman's daughter to ask for her opinion, but the daughter forbade cohabitation on the grounds that her mother always loved her husband, that faithful marriage meant everything to her, and that her cohabitation now would make a mockery of a lifetime of fidelity. In the end, the two were not allowed to cohabit.

Was this not a case in which the woman with dementia was being exploited by the other resident of the nursing home because she clearly could not meaningfully consent to sex? It would seem so. And what would have happened if she had regained enough insight to realize that the man she was sleeping with was not her late husband? What counts as hedonic happiness and appears beneficial in the pure present may on a deeper level disrespect the identity of the self over the course of a lifetime, and the deep-seated values that have shaped a person's life journey.

When dealing with deeply forgetful people and making decisions regarding their care, it is always important to realize that there is no real divide between the "then" self and the "now" self. Only in the very advanced stage of the disease can we speak more of a loss of continuity with the past in the person with dementia, although even at this point, far into the illness experience, all deeply forgetful people will have moments of insight and remembering. I have witnessed persons with advanced dementia who have had moments of insight into the identity of a loved one who has simply been sitting by the bedside and reminiscing about the past. In one case, a man who had not spoken for several months seemed to move his eyes toward two old friends who were chatting about the trio's college days. As the old friends got up to leave, the patient suddenly responded with "good times."

Additional Core Values in Caregiver Ethics

The two key values for caregiver ethics are human dignity and care. But there are other values we should be explicit about:

1. Inclusion. Diminished intellect and memory does not make any human being something less than a full "person"—in contrast to what numerous philosophers term "nonpersons," a humiliating language of "othering" rooted in both implicit and often explicit bias. A cognitively disabled person is a feeling, receptive, expressive, and experiencing human being with tastes and preferences. Simply being consciously aware of the surrounding world—from the singing of the birds to the colors of fall leaves to the smells of a kitchen—is grounds for human equality. Impaired intellect does not demote anyone

from the family of humanity. Distinctions between "persons" and "nonpersons" are unfairly biased, with the exception of those who are whole-brain dead, anencephalic (with only a brain stem), or clearly diagnosed to be in a persistent vegetative state with no brain activity outside of the brain stem. In other words, the only line of meaningful moral demarcation is between those who are conscious and those who are not.

2. Partialities. Every conscious person is someone's child, sibling, or parent who is part of an interpersonal relational nexus that involves interdependence, vulnerability, and caregiving with kindness. These relationships generate responsibilities that are stronger than responsibilities to distant others, although the latter are also important and not to be lost sight of. While caregivers must tend to loved ones immediately in front of them they should still lean outward in appreciation of the needs of all people with compassionate intention. But special relationships between the near and dear (family and friends) do have moral weight and special pull. Impartial aspects of caregiver ethics center on an activism within a community of care that promotes justice for this entire constituency of deeply forgetful people and caregivers. Connections create responsibilities. Dependency and related caregiving have not been a priority of mainstream philosophers.

3. Sustainability. A caregiver must know how to care for themselves through self-regulation, self-awareness, balance, perhaps meditational practice, exercise, self-compassion, and a willingness to relinquish caregiving to others rather than be overwhelmed. The ethics of care is not the unsustainable embrace of self-immolation and radical self-sacrifice. We must do everything possible to prevent caregiver burnout, and that requires justice in the provision of supportive resources. Respite care must be made available as an ethical imperative to enable caregivers to flourish. A just society is one in which caregiver flourishing is the hallmark of moral quality.

4. Situationalism. The ethics of care makes choices based on particular relationships and circumstances. Sure, it is good to have some mid-level principles like maximize benefits and minimize harms in one's back pockets, and the comparison of cases (casuistry) as well. But caregivers respond to circumstances and needs with improvisational innovation. *They do what is caring.*

5. Listening. Caregiving has been the province mostly of people who have been less listened to historically, primarily women, who more often than not have been the ones who serve others as personal attendants, nurses, nurses' aides, grade-school teachers, wives, mothers, daughters-in-law, and so forth. To make caregiving the very center of an ethical philosophy (Kittay 2019) is a complete contrast with the historically male-dominated theories that diminish the importance of special caring relationships and give them no attention. The ethics of care seeks to awaken us from dogmatic focus on independent autonomous individuals rather than on relationship, dependency, and connectivity in their embodied existence (Kittay 2019, 171). Care is gravitational in the sense that closer relationships take precedence, like the pull between planets, and it is here that we need to focus our deep moral analysis.

6. Connectivity. Philosopher Kittay, widely considered to be the world's leading feminist ethicist of care and with whom I have had the honor of interacting at Stony Brook University, writes, "Modern theories of ethics begin with independent autonomous individuals as moral agents in rational pursuit of their own good. . . . An Ethics of Care begins with embodied selves who are regarded as inextricably connected to other embodied selves" (Kittay 2019, 173). The ethics of care focuses on the cultivation of interpersonal relationships as good: "Care . . . is also a virtue to be cultivated. . . . the degree to which the caregiver must become enmeshed . . . in another's needs in order to adequately meet those needs varies with

both the urgency and extent of the other's dependency and with the degree to which one has cultivated the virtue of care" (Kittay 2019, 172).

Kittay writes: "Ethical theories within a liberal tradition stress the importance of people being able to live their lives according to their own lights. . . . An Ethics of Care stresses, first of all, the concern for the well-being (or flourishing) of a person *for their own sake* and the moral importance of enabling each one to flourish" (Kittay 2019, 177).

The moral values that are important to women were revealed in the early 1980s when psychologist Lawrence Kohlberg interviewed men and boys to delineate moral maturation, an evolution in the personal development of ethical behavior or consciousness. This study of males revealed an evolution from abiding by the law, to working for the greatest good of all. The work, and its clearly male-dominated illustration of moral maturation, gave psychologist Carol Gilligan insight into the bias of ethical studies. In response, Gilligan replicated the intention of the inquiry but focused instead on studying women and girls and ethical choices. Her study revealed significant distinctions in how females determine the right action: women and girls showed consideration for how action would impact surrounding people, relationships, and future outcomes.

————

Caregivers need an ethic that actually focuses on providing care—on the cultivation of relationships, on noticing expressions of selfhood, on kindness, and on concrete needs—that leaves no one behind, particularly the disabled and underserved who are so often marginalized by historical Western thought and practice. We need to consider the larger picture of addressing the needs and legitimate wants as a caregiver would understand them. The tools for the caregiver's moral deliberation are not neatly packaged moral principles, since her circumstances are too complex for that: to a large extent, caregivers care and do what seems fitting in the particular situation.

The ethics of care, and specifically Alzheimer's care, gets to questions that other theories tend to neglect as uninteresting, perhaps because the ethics of care is the product of women philosophers, most of whom are themselves caregivers performing the concrete actions of caring for children, spouse, and parents. This ethics of care addresses the considerations that someone tending to a deeply forgetful person (or a child, someone with developmental disabilities, or for that matter anyone who becomes highly dependent in their human frailty) wants to discuss at a wise and practical level. The questions an ethics of care addresses are to be primarily those identified by caregivers themselves.

Breaking Free from Hypercognitive Personhood

I have studied with some great philosophers and theologians at several universities, most notably the University of Chicago. Looking back on my years as a student and faculty member, I cannot recall a single line on any course syllabus that included the word "caregiving"—until I came to Stony Brook and met the great feminist philosopher of care Eva Kittay. Thus, I transitioned long ago into medical education and work with the Alzheimer's community to save my soul, especially as I realized that according to the dominant hypercognitive and hyper-rational definitions of personhood, Grandma Post and people like her could only have a vanishingly low moral standing and could therefore be easily expendable.

Through working with deeply forgetful people and their caregivers I have been able to break free of the influence of hypercognitive philosophers and the mainstream bioethicists who espouse exclusionary hypercognitive values (Post 1995b) and see little to do with deeply forgetful people other than somehow euthanize them. I have been troubled by this approach since the early 1990s when I developed "hypercognitive" as a term crucial of this narrowing. Bioethicists are uninterested in the emotional, relational, aesthetic, creative, and spiritual aspects of continuing self-identity in deeply forgetful people. Their interest is in rational capacity for meaningful decision making.

In her magnum opus *Learning from My Daughter: The Value and Care of Disabled Minds* (2019), Kittay develops a compelling criticism of philosophers who have taken no interest in examining the meaning and lives of children with cognitive developmental disabilities or the mother-child relationship involved, other than to dismiss such children as still "human" in some general sense, but not real "persons" of equal worth, dignity, and rights. Kittay's adult daughter Sesha cannot speak and is entirely dependent, but she intensely enjoys music, can beam love and enjoys giving hugs, but according to certain philosophers such people are incapable of deep personal relations, achievement, and the attainment of knowledge. A number of these philosophers (Peter Singer, for instance) have explicitly refused to spend time with Sesha or people like her, displaying a lack of curiosity about her ability to experience joy and bring joy to those around her. In other words, arrogance precludes knowledge of the cognitively imperiled, though thankfully the philosopher Alasdair MacIntyre is one exception (Post 2000). Kittay describes herself as remaining a philosopher with some difficulty, but she persists to challenge her professional peers. She wants the thick and rich description of people like Sesha to be a major project for philosophers, as it should be (Kittay 2019, xxi).

Western philosophers make too much of intellectual dexterity. The great Stoic philosophers did much to elevate our universal human moral standing by emphasizing the spark of reason (*logos*) in us all. This is, however, an arrogant view in the sense that it makes the worth of a human being entirely dependent on rationality, and then gives too much power to the reasonable. From the Stoics and onward without interruption to Kant, Locke, and modern bioethics we find the rude assertion that the major criterion for "moral membership" is reason—and this tends to include only the intelligent members of the protected community. We easily demean those whose memory has dissipated by treating them with indifference or even with cruelty. Theologian Reinhold Niebuhr wrote of the ancient Stoic philosophical tradition: "Since the divine principle is reason, the logic of Stoicism tends to include only the intelligent in the divine community. An aristocratic condescension, therefore, corrupts Stoic universalism" (Niebuhr 1956). As intellectual heirs of the Stoics, most philosophers show no interest in those who have lost the power of reason and who in the process may actually reveal the things in life and human interaction that are more important than reason (Post 2000).

The rationality that philosophers select for moral consideration is generally limited to one property: they define rationality procedurally as an ability to do certain things, such as to act consistently based on clear thinking, arrive at decisions by deliberation, envisage a future for oneself, and so forth. But, in fact, rather few of us live our lives with consistent rationality (Zagzebski 2001). We act on emotion, intuition, impulse, and the like. We pass through periods of considerable irrationality due to variations in mood. Rationality as the capacity to make decisions is not morally important. It is rationality as a source of self-identity that matters—who we are rather than how we proceed. And in this sense, the deeply forgetful can be surprising.

Our task as caregivers and advocates is to remind persons with dementia of their continuing self-identity, of who they are. In other words, our task is to preserve identity, rather than to deny it. It is for this reason that many units for the deeply forgetful in nursing homes will post biographical sketches on the doors of residents, or family members will remind a loved one of events and people who have been meaningful along their life's journey.

How can we encounter the deeply forgetful outside the strictures of hypercognitive ideologies? How can we bear witness to the meaning of these lives, and create a culture where all are welcomed and celebrated regardless of cognitive limits and vulnerability? Giving affected individuals a public voice early on in the progression of their memory loss and allowing them to speak for themselves will help. Perhaps more caregivers need to tell the story of why they value their loved ones despite cognitive deficits.

Rationality is too severe a criterion for moral standing. The fitting moral response to people with dementia is to enlarge our sense of human worth to counter an exclusionary emphasis on the importance of rationality, efficient use of time and energy, ability to control distracting impulses, thrift, economic success, self-reliance, self-control, "language advantage," and the like. The perils of forgetfulness are especially evident in a culture like our own, which promotes independence and economic productivity—one that so values intellect, memory, and self-control. Particularly in this contradictory cultural context, we need to bear in mind that emotional, relational, aesthetic, creative, olfactory, spiritual, and symbolic well-being are possible for people with progressive dementia.

Is a Deeply Forgetful Person a Person? Yes.

"Personhood" afforded to the intelligent becomes a dangerous exclusionary term. Technically, *persona* in Latin refers to an actor's mask.
It has to do with the roles we play in the theater of life. The philosophers of personhood seem to state that if we do not exhibit
the persona dictated by their attitudes as modern liberal intellectuals, we count for less. Some very astute philosophers, such as Ber-
nard Williams (1973), have pointed out the varied definitions of personhood, and Williams is skeptical about the ability of personhood
theories to do any genuine moral work in the real world of human
experience. Without delving into this literature, suffice it to state
that philosophers have arrived at no consensus as to what constitutes personhood. Peter Singer does list "indicators of personhood":
"self-awareness, self-control, a sense of the future, a sense of the past,
the capacity to relate to others, concern for others, communication,
and curiosity" (Singer 1993, 86). Based on these criteria, would anyone really qualify consistently, let alone a deeply forgetful person?

As Jenny Teichman argues regarding "personhood" theories, the
restricted definition of person "has the consequence that some people are not persons and is therefore rather similar to the doctrine
that only white Anglo-Saxon Protestants really matter" (Teichman
1985, 181). Better to quicken the spirit of beneficence toward mentally
weakened persons than to undermine it. Historically, this orientation
toward beneficence is related to a shift in the moral tone of Western
civilization, which now sympathizes with and even gives preference
to the vulnerable and weak, making beneficent service the highest
virtue.

The appropriate response to the increasing incidence of dementia in our
aging society is to come closer and learn so as to expand our sense of human

worth, thereby countering an exclusionary emphasis on rationality, efficient use of time and energy, ability to control distracting impulses, thrift, economic success, self-reliance, "language advantage," and the like.

Caring Communication

There are about thirty people on a care unit called "the schmooze room," which is nicely designed and incorporates all the latest environmental details to allow residents ambulation and freedom without much fear of a fall. It is easy for residents to walk out into a fenced outdoor area, sit down, and enjoy nature. The schmooze room is attached to the unit and easily accessible. It is in such places that deeply forgetful people can reveal to outsiders who they are, what they value, and how we can extend ourselves to them as "differently abled."

Anyone who derides deeply forgetful people as "gone" should spend a few days in this schmooze room. It is a square space about thirty feet by thirty feet containing comfortable, reclining vinyl couches in greens and blues, but wheelchairs are also welcome if individuals use them. The door to the room is closed; soft meditational music plays in the background, and the scent of lavender hovers in the air. The soft green lights are dimmed—green because social psychologists have long noted the color's calming effects. About eight people are in the room at any one time, and different groups rotate in and out, each spending about an hour there. After a half hour of relaxation, the background music fades away and it is time for personalized iPod musical interventions, which are offered at least once a day for each resident.

Following the lead of Dan Cohen's internationally renowned Music and Memory program, an earphone headset attached to an iPod is placed on the resident, who then listens for a while to deeply meaningful music that they loved earlier in life and identified with. Family members enjoy helping to choose this music as only they can do, since they are so familiar with their loved one's preferences. As they listen, residents' faces light up with a wide smile, and most of them start to move their bodies in time to the music, or at least tap their feet a bit as they rest on the recliner. Most will also begin to hum or sing along or conduct with their hands. Through this process they get back in touch with who they still are, and after ten minutes or so the headphones are gently removed.

Then they are especially likely to respond to a simply phrased question asked in an affirming voice, such as "So, do you like the Beatles?" or "Do you just love that Brubeck jazz?" They usually respond (in an estimated 70 percent of cases) with comments such as "Oh, that's so beautiful," or "Oh, I feel so happy," or "Thank you, thank you, thank you." Then the background music comes back on for a while.

If a family member is visiting the "schmooze room" they are inspired, because they see that even at this advanced stage their loved one can still connect with their favorite music and will frequently respond to them and call them by name for a minute or two right after the headphones are removed. Then the resident will calmly fade back into deep forgetfulness and be relatively tranquil. This is also a great way to involve family members in care, not only because they see that "Grandma is really still there, wow!" but because it is a refreshingly contemplative experience for them to simply sit for a while in the quietly affective presence of their loved one.

A woman named Sonia works with the deeply forgetful people in the schmooze room. She offers shoulder and foot massages, and the offer is almost uniformly well received, but Sonia always begins with a quiet question, "Hi, Jim, would you like a little massage on your shoulders?" An answer may not come, and it is still fine to proceed, but at least the question was asked, with the possibility that it might elicit a response.

Sonia has a degree in gerontology and counseling, so she finds working with these older adults highly meaningful, and she also connects really well with the residents' family members. She describes her work as a calling or vocation. She gets a half-decent salary—nothing great, although recently she had gotten a raise and was grateful for it. But she quoted the great writer of the 1920s, Kahlil Gibran, who said that "work is love made visible," "or at least," she added, "it should be. For me, this is so meaningful, and I never feel empty inside for a moment."

In the schmooze room I saw love at work and miracles happening every moment, and response effects that seemed to bring deeply forgetful people into view, revealing who they always were and who they still are and always will be. None of them are on any kind of medication for Alzheimer's because at this point the available medications, already relatively useless even early on, are especially pointless. In any case, there is absolutely no medicine that can manifest these miracles of tender loving care.

Can We Learn to Communicate?

Sonia shared with me what she had learned about the importance of developing special techniques for communicating with people with dementia in the hope of drawing them out. She studies these techniques with care and practices them daily. This is an area of particular research for one of my old friends from Case Western days, Daniele "Danny" Ripich (1990). She and nurse gerontologist May Wykle (1990) were always busy designing techniques for enhanced communication between nurse's aides and people with Alzheimer's, and I learned much from both of them. Their seven-step program uses the acronym FOCUSED to identify the major elements necessary for the maintenance of communication and is based on an interactive discourse model of conversational exchanges.

The strategies used to achieve and maintain FOCUSED communication with Alzheimer's-affected individuals are:

F   Face to face
1. Face the person directly.
2. Attract the person's attention with a calm statement, calling them by name.
3. Maintain eye contact.

O   Orientation
1. Repeat sentences exactly.
2. Give the person time to comprehend what you say and be patient.

C   Continuity
1. Continue the same topic of conversation for as long as possible.
2. Prepare the person if a new topic must be introduced.

U   Unsticking
1. Help the person become "unstuck" when he or she uses a word incorrectly by suggesting the correct or missing word.
2. Repeat the person's sentence using the correct or missing word.
3. Ask, "Do you mean . . . ?"

S   Structure
1. Structure your questions to give the person a choice of response. For example, "Would you like tomato soup or autumn squash?"
2. Provide only two or three options at a time.
3. Provide options that the person would like as you have known them.

E   Exchange

1. Begin conversations with pleasant topics.
2. Ask easy questions that the person can answer.
3. Give the person clues as to how to answer.

D   Direct

1. Keep sentences short, simple, and direct (subject, verb, object).
2. Use and repeat nouns rather than pronouns.
3. Use hand signals, pictures, and facial expressions.

Nonadversarial and noncorrective caregiving, coupled with thoughtful methods of communication, will enhance the emotional well-being of dementia-affected individuals and limit their sense of isolation (Sabat 1994; Sabat and Cagigas 1997).

It is in very advanced dementia, when meaningful verbal communication is assumed to be over and done with, that other communicative methods are of perhaps the greatest importance. The communication we establish with a newborn through emotional warmth and touch can also be extended to people with Alzheimer's as a standard of care. These people can be reassured that someone is with them in solidarity by the simple, solicitous act of touching a shoulder. This form of care is crucially important for their well-being and identifies a core of humanness in both self and other. One act of discourse is extending a hand; another is using a tone of voice that reassures the other person. This is the sort of basic act that makes possible resurrection of a sort—the resurrection of a sense of self in the person we are reaching out to.

Conclusions

In the tenth book of his *Confessions*, Augustine wrote these elegant words about the majesty of memory—lines that would echo over the centuries in the Western intellectual tradition and inspire many other great thinkers:

> All this goes on inside me, in the vast cloisters of my memory. In it are the sky, the earth, and the sea, ready at my summons, together with everything that I have ever perceived in them by my senses, except the things which I have forgotten. In it I meet myself as well. I remember myself and what I have done, when and where I did it, and the state of my mind at the time. In my memory, too, are all the events that I remember, whether they are things that have happened to me or things that I have heard from others. (Augustine 1961, x, 8)

Augustine held memory in awe, as though through it he were touching the mysteries of the infinite soul. He argues that memory was an activity of the soul, and he did not think that the deterioration of any organ, including the brain, could erase it.

I do not vouch for a nonmaterial soul or memory being housed therein, but memory is a wondrous power that makes our life narratives possible. However, caregivers teach us that the dignity of a deeply forgetful person is always there, even when memory greatly fades while we remain open to surprises and expressions of those life narratives that come to the surface in so many small and wondrous ways.

Jan experienced peace in light snowfall, in the quiet of natural beauty, and she felt a certain spirituality of joy. As I recall Jan, there was a certain radiance about her that seemed to be as valuable as the keen memory she once had. Seeing this radiance and joy in Jan is, finally, the essence of respect and the basis of care.

6

Respecting the Preferences of Deeply Forgetful People in Health Care and Research

Stephen G. Post, PhD, and Phyllis Migdal, MD, MA

This chapter provides a special focus on clinical ethical decision making and the extent to which deeply forgetful people can contribute to that decision making. Because the topic is so central to our daily clinical ethical consultations, it is worthy of separate attention, although it is discussed quite differently in chapters three and five. Here the focus is on the procedural aspects of capacity determination, and on who exactly should be making these decisions.

The decisional capacities of those with dementia should be respected. As the condition progresses, preferences will generally be more apparent in the various forms of response to specific activities of daily living rather than in health care decisions that are complex conceptually and require stable comprehension of information over time. We will first address daily living and then turn to health care decisions.

Respecting remaining capacities in deeply forgetful people (Post 2000) is more likely when stigmatizing language (like "already gone," "half dead," "a husk") is rejected. We need to *notice* continuity of self-hood despite forgetfulness. A "noticer" picks up on indicators of self-identity and can display a gentle curiosity about preferences.

Some deeply forgetful people, even when encouraged, will display noninvolvement and be passive recipients of care; some will engage in a reassuring exchange of information; some will be able to engage in real shared decision making; and some will still be able to express relatively independent decisions. We can expect great variability (Smebye, Kirkevold, and Engedal 2012).

Why make efforts to respect decisional capacity? Because deeply forgetful people, in the mild and moderate phases certainly, but also beyond into severe dementia, do have subjectivity and value their dignity; allowing the expression of their subjective experience and preference is to respect them and to be kind rather than dismissive. Research indicates that those with mild or moderate dementia can be very clear about just how important being respected is to them and how much having a sense of choice matters to their well-being (Ises et al. 2016).

Everyday Preferences

When it comes to everyday preferences in the present moment, any discussion about "then" and "now" selves only diverts attention from what is much more important in this domain, namely, the *whole underlying self who is in this moment attempting to convey preferences* about small gratifications that come to loom large (Koppelman 2002). As possibilities for pleasure and meaning erode, minor gratifications grow in significance. By doing what we can to include and engage deeply forgetful people at this level, we contribute to their quality of life emotionally and relationally, and to their enjoyment of the world around them. While the capacity of deeply forgetful people to express everyday preferences is understandably not discussed in medical ethics literature, it certainly is discussed and researched in studies on caregiving. Deeply forgetful people value opportunities to be involved in choice to the extent they can, and such involvement can be strongly determinative of well-being (Daly, Bunn, and Goodman 2018).

Caregivers may think of communicating with deeply forgetful people as a special gift and a privilege. When they encounter the intense joy in singing a meaningful song with a loved one, or when they recite a poem together at an "Alzheimer's poet" session, or when caregiver and loved one hug an Alzheimer's dog, we are reminded of what really matters in life.

Health Care Decisions

Regarding health care decisions, those who have an early diagnosis of progressive dementia will find solace in the assurance that their wishes will be reasonably well honored as they eventually decline. These previously expressed wishes of the "then" self should be respected because the "then" self is always also the "now" self, and any bifurcation is doubtful. Wishes as expressed before decline through advance directives should be taken seriously because they commemorate the dignity of choice. These preferences may pertain to the use or non-use of artificial nutrition and hydration, CPR, continued use of insulin for diabetes, antibiotics in case of infection, treatment for chronic heart conditions, and so forth. Let us err on the side of honoring these wishes, be they expressed in a living will, attached to a durable power of attorney form, or verbally expressed to family members. Someone may state that they would never want to have a feeding tube placed should they develop severe dementia and be unable to swallow, or to be treated with chemotherapy should a tumor return. This sort of extension of autonomy is a matter of right, and clearly no one should be forced to die with tubes placed here and there.

Having dementia does not rule out significant ongoing involvement in health care decision making. Decisions are going to be shared or relational with caregivers because deeply forgetful people depend heavily on others in all things, medical decisions included. Decisions tend to be triadic, involving the person with dementia, the caregiver who notices preferences and expressed wishes more closely due to past experience with the affected individual, and the involved health care provider. As dementia progresses the individual may no longer be the one to lead the decision making, but that individual can participate quite significantly and later can at least express meaningful dissent that is worthy of serious consideration.

The diagnosis of dementia necessarily encompasses consideration of decision-making capacity in a way not initially considered for persons with other newly diagnosed medical illnesses. Underlying the general concept of autonomy is the question "Does this individual have the capacity to make and provide informed consent for medical decisions?" The requirements necessary for capacity to participate in medical decision making and informed consent remain a central topic of concern to the essential care triad (Stubbe 2017).

An important survey of Americans reported that despite agreement about the value of having conversations early in the diagnosis of life-threatening illnesses, the majority of individuals stated that their end-of-life wishes were not discussed (Goodman 2014). Goodman, cofounder of "The Conversation Project" (an organization that focuses on engaging in conversations about end-of-life wishes early in an illness), believes in the value of these discussions early in the diagnosis of dementia, concluding, "It's always too soon until it's too late" (Goodman 2014). Advantages associated with end-of-life discussions also spill over to family members as less anxiety, stress, and depression are reported by relatives (Detering et al. 2010; Wright et al. 2008). For this reason, early assessment and (appropriately) frequent evaluation of capacity needs to be addressed when the diagnosis of dementia is made.

In order to maintain individual self-determination and dignity an understanding of the person's values and priorities is key. Practicing surgeon and author of *Being Mortal* Atul Gawande urges health care providers to understand what an individual values and to acknowledge that "sometimes we can offer cure, sometimes only a salve, sometimes not even that. But whatever we can offer, our interventions, and the risks and sacrifices they entail, are justified only if they serve the larger aims of a person's life" (Gawande 2014, 260).

Significant concern arises about the loss of autonomy and the loss of one's enduring self upon diagnosis of dementia. Briefly, *capacity* is distinguished from *competency*, which is a legal term that refers to the ability to make decisions as determined in court. Capacity pertains to a specific task and is determined in the clinical environment by clinicians and/or the clinical team. Capacity is determined for some specified decision, but not for all decisions. Competency is only determined by the courts, and while it can be focused on one area of decision making but not others, it can also be determined globally for all decisions. Thus, an individual may be declared incompetent by a court to make their own financial decisions yet still competent to make medical choices, or else incompetent in a general sense. This distinction is an important one especially for persons with dementia (Leo 1999). Capacity is a situational evaluation operationalized in the clinical setting and as such assessments need to be fluid, considered frequently and on a timely basis surrounding a particular decision (Hedge and Ellajosyula 2016).

Many people with less severe dementia can be surprisingly consistent when it comes to health care decisions; their capacity should be assessed with the usual four elements in view:

1. Understanding of relevant information for this specific decision at hand

2. Appreciation of the significance of the decision

3. Ability to consider alternatives

4. Reasonably apparent and *stable* expression of choice

We add the word "stable" above because for this population, an individual might sound quite capable until a minute later they respond to the same question in exactly the opposite way. In other words, they have no consistency over time because they forget what they thought or said in the preceding moments. This can be quite surprising—but not to anyone who is familiar with deeply forgetful people.

Authenticity in making decisions about capacity implies that "capacity assessments are recognized inherently to involve judgments of value concerning the situated embodied agent as well as the factual matters involving cognitive functions" (Hughes 2014, 106; Barstow, Shahan, and Roberts 2018). Hughes goes on to further elucidate that the assessment of capacity is the appreciation that "we are not just cognitive computational machines. We are, amongst other things, emotional, evaluative and volitional creatures too; and our decision-making reflects our complex make-up" (Hughes 2014, 97). It is recognized that self-determination and authenticity are entwined, that when self-determination is no longer an option surrogate decision making is viewed as the exercise of the moral value of autonomy.

Clarifying the underlying moral and ethical responsibilities that providers, caregivers, and persons with dementia have regarding the concept of autonomy and how the conceptualization of autonomy assists in maintaining dignity and well-being provides a framework for approaching autonomy in the deeply forgetful. Post and colleagues outline a refocusing of empathy and compassion as necessary components for optimal care of patients. Compassionate care is defined as "a deep response to suffering at the affective level and appropriate action to relieve it" (Post et al. 2014, 875). In rethinking the concept of autonomy in patients with dementia, a focus on compassionate autonomy is considered and assumes initiative to respond in ways that continue to uphold their autonomy. Embracing the development, continuation, and enhancement of relationships in the interactions of the essential care triad focuses decision making along a continuum that inevitably shifts from the person with dementia to the caregiver(s) as the disease progresses. The concept of compassionate autonomy sets the expectation that decision making remains centralized around the values and the well-being of the patient even as cognition declines and the locus of decision making changes.

The importance of advance directives was made clear in chapter three, but it bears repeating that such directives provide an opportunity for the intact self to outline their personal values and vision of care when the disease progresses and they become unable to make complex, informed decisions. A health care proxy names a trusted family member or friend as their health care agent when the individual lacks decision-making capacity. Ideally this agent has had conversations that explicate not just what the person with dementia may want done in certain situations, for example tube-feeding placement or DNR status, but also what their loved one valued, how their life has had meaning, and what they have considered a "good life." If advance directives were not completed or a health care agent was not named prior to the loss of decision-making capacity, then surrogate decision makers such as family or a close friend are generally called upon to make medical treatment decisions.

Recalling the adage "It's always too soon until it's too late," the health care provider can also initiate conversations to encourage the use of advance directives and to develop an understanding of their patient to enhance cohesiveness within the essential care triad (Jensen and Inker 2014). Autonomy is inherently grounded in authenticity as it is perceived as the capacity to be a particular self, true to the concept of one's beliefs and values, or "doing things in a way that is authentic to the person" (Brudney 2009, 32). Conversations early in the diagnosis between the involved triad of care can establish greater confidence that the wishes of the person with dementia are being honored by being faithful to the individual's personality and values, upholding their dignity and autonomy even when the arena of autonomy shifts to other decision makers.

Such discussions and advance directives enable substituted judgment, which refers to decision making for the person who lacks capacity based upon the known preferences of the patient, either as expressed in advance directives or through conversation. In contrast, decisions on their behalf are based on the best-interest standard.

Clinical ethical decision making is grounded in four principles, including autonomy (self-determination), beneficence, nonmaleficence, and justice. Though equally valued there may be situations where one of the principles is given stronger priority. For example, as dementia progresses priority may shift away from personal autonomy toward beneficence or nonmaleficence, due to the (re)-assessment of capacity. While the person with dementia may still be involved in discussion, choices may need to be narrowed and weight redistributed to the health care agent or surrogate decision maker with guidance concerning the proportionality of risks and benefits by the health care provider. Beneficence, defined as "the moral obligation to act for the benefit of others" or taking actions to improve the health and well-being of others (Beauchamp and Childress 2013, 203), is further actualized through upholding self-determination by aligning surrogate decision making with the patient's own view of a life well-lived.

Reconceptualization: Compassionate Autonomy

This reconceptualization of autonomy in the deeply forgetful toward a model of compassionate autonomy expands upon the four principles approach. Compassion-fostering action enables autonomy to be viewed along a spectrum that at extreme ends includes self-determination and at the opposite end decision making by others. Essential to the concept of compassionate autonomy is that it is grounded in relationships and may be expressed along a continuum that maintains dignity and authenticity based on present capacity assessments of persons with dementia. Even as capacity for self-determination declines, the expression of autonomy can be deemed appropriate and authentic when provided by others within this framework.

Compassionate autonomy recognizes the contribution of the model of relationship-centered care (RCC) and the theory of care ethics as its practical and moral foundation. At its heart RCC encompasses the understanding of the value of health within a network of interpersonal meaning and "[recognizes] that the nature and quality of relationships are central to health care and the broader health care delivery system" (Beach and Inui 2006, S3). Included in the guiding principles of RCC is the understanding of the centrality of relationships in several areas, namely,

1. that relationships in health care ought to include the personhood of the participants,
2. that affect and emotion are important components of these relationships,

3. that all health care relationships occur in the context of recip-
rocal influence, and

4. that the formation and maintenance of genuine relationships
in health care is morally valuable (Beach and Inui 2006, S3).

RCC provides the scaffolding to commit to early conversations between the essential care triad to gain further insight into the important decisions that inevitably need to be addressed in persons with
dementia and may increase the comfort of the caregivers and health
care providers for having these conversations early on.

Care ethics extends the centrality of relationships to fully realize autonomy (Verkerk 2001). Conceiving autonomy as solely independent isolates decision making within a vacuum not influenced by
others; seldom are decisions made this way. Care ethics "stresses that
autonomy as a moral capacity can only be developed in relation to
others" (Verkerk 2001, 292). It is within this relationship-based framework of autonomy that Verkerk developed the concept of relational
autonomy. As such, principles of RCC are synergistic with the concept of relational autonomy and allow practical and morally sound
expression of autonomy in the deeply forgetful.

Compassionate autonomy furthers the understanding of decision
making in persons with dementia such that self-determination may
be expressed along a continuum that maintains dignity and authenticity, values inherently important to persons with dementia. Even
as capacity for self-determination declines the expression of autonomy can be deemed appropriate when provided by others within this
framework (Reed, Carson, and Gibb 2017). Compassionate autonomy
accounts for the necessarily relationally based decision-making process and elucidates the motivation to act that remains faithful to the
dignity and autonomy of the deeply forgetful.

See a Lawyer

Caregivers and the deeply forgetful person they care for are a dyad. Therefore, the caregiver will be essential in making medical shared decisions with a loved one. In clinical ethical practice, cases involving deeply forgetful people are often vexing and complex with no easy answers. It is important for people with a diagnosis of dementia to see a lawyer or go online and file a durable power of attorney for health care, stating who they want making medical decisions on their behalf should they no longer be able to. This way the caregiver can be a clearly designated and empowered advocate for a loved one.

In the case described below, a person named Mr. Key has, by formally filing a living will and durable power of attorney for health care, indicated that Mrs. Key is his legal "agent." It should be noted that Mr. Key might have selected a friend or someone else who knows him well and whom he trusts instead of a family member. He might simply have wanted to unburden his family from having to make decisions. While Mr. Key had cognitive capacity he was always his own "agent" and could make his decisions in compassionate relational autonomy with (presumably) Mrs. Key by his side.

Had Mr. Key not indicated his legal agent, decision making would fall to family surrogates, who by virtue of being family members have legal authority by most state statutes. The authority would rest with the spouse first, but with no spouse remaining, authority would rest with adult children, and then with siblings. While Mrs. Key would then have the surrogate authority to make decisions, she would likely have engaged with the family so as to get everyone on the same page (if possible). This is important in order to avoid any legacy of resentment on the part of those who might disagree with her. *Consensus is helpful and recommended,* but sometimes consensus is impossible to achieve. Regardless, Mrs. Key has the final word.

The following is a composite de-identified case of Mr. Key, as presented to medical students at Stony Brook School of Medicine, although here it is revised and abridged.

CASE STUDY. John Key is a sixty-six-year-old man admitted to this hospital about one month ago for third-degree burns of his chest and right arm. Mr. Key has lived at a nursing home since a stroke in 2000 left him with a right hemiparesis. He also suffers from some degree of progressive dementia, although he can carry on a conversation and take care of himself. His past medical history includes coronary artery disease, diabetes, and alcohol abuse. He was smoking his pipe in the nursing home when evidently a falling ember from the pipe ignited his shirt.

Mr. Key's burns required a number of surgeries but have now essentially healed. He suffered from a bout of pneumonia; this cleared, but he is currently being treated for a presumed blood infection (sepsis). About two weeks ago the patient developed acute renal failure, presumptively secondary to acute tubular necrosis (ATN). As a result of multiple acute medical problems superimposed on chronic dementia, the patient was virtually unresponsive; he clearly lacked decision-making capacity. When ATN developed, a family conference was held with Dr. Jacobs, and they made the decision not to begin dialysis, but rather take a "comfort care only" approach. Though Mr. Key was expected to die imminently, he lingered for a week and began showing signs of renal improvement, such as increased urine output. At this point another family conference was held. Agreeing with Dr. Jacobs's strong recommendation, the patient's wife, Mrs. Key, somewhat reluctantly agreed to a one-week trial of continuous venous-venous hemodialysis (CVVHD); they would then meet and discuss further treatment decisions. However, the next day Mrs. Key came into the hospital with Mr. Key's advance directive and asked that dialysis be stopped. The advance directive, a written living will, and health care proxy form listed four conditions under which Mr. Key would not like life-prolonging treatment to continue.

At this point, Mrs. Key asked for a clinical ethics consult. Two ethics consultants met with Dr. Jacobs, along with the University Hospital patient advocate, a chaplain, the nurse unit manager, the burn fellow, and other members of the nursing staff. After discussing the issues to get the consulting team oriented, the group invited the patient's wife, their son and daughter-in-law, and the patient's brother to a meeting to discuss their concerns.

It is clear that Dr. Jacobs strongly favors continued dialysis. He believes that there is a reasonable chance that Mr. Key's ATN will improve and that he can be restored to his pre-morbid condition. Dr. Jacobs had acceded to the family's original decision against continuing dialysis, but he believes Mr. Key's increased urine output and failure to die promptly are evidence that he has a real chance to recover from the immediate crisis. He presents this improved outlook to the family with the intention of having them change their decision. An infectious disease physician, on the other hand, paints a very grim picture of Mr. Key's prognosis. No one is willing to give a quantitative estimate for Mr. Key's survival and neurological improvement. Since ATN is often reversible, a trial of dialysis to "tide him over" appears reasonable. However, his poor nutritional status and possible septicemia decrease his chances.

It is also clear that the family has struggled mightily with decisions about Mr. Key's medical care. Mrs. Key is fatigued and overwhelmed. The family members present are sensitive to and supportive of one another. They describe the process over the last month as being a "yo-yo"—at times it looks like Mr. Key will die, then suddenly it appears as if he might recover, then the sequence occurs again. This is emotionally exhausting. They want to do the best thing, but it is not clear to them whether they are merely prolonging Mr. Key's dying or really giving him a chance to live.

Dr. Jacobs and the staff appear to be sensitive to Mrs. Key and other family members and are acknowledging their role as decision makers. Mrs. Key has been mostly passive in the sense that she goes along with all recommended treatments on the basis of her belief that Mr. Key would do so, except when his advance directive appears to specify otherwise. Her daughter (not present) evidently does not agree with this approach and has made provocative comments about the hospital "keeping him alive for no reason." The son and brother seem to understand the emotional complexities of the situation, although it appears that the brother at least leans toward terminating life support. Dr. Jacobs strongly supports aggressive care and has consciously tried to influence Mrs. Key to continue treatment.

Mrs. Key has consistently indicated that her husband was a fighter and that he would probably keep fighting to recover, even against the odds. Dr. Jacobs and the medical staff do not believe that Mr. Key's clinical condition meets any of the criteria specified in his advance directive under which he would like care withdrawn. However, the advance directive also specifies that Mrs. Key can make any and all decisions regarding his care. She has recently indicated that "he wouldn't want to live like this."

Mr. Key's written living will and health care proxy form reads as follows:

> If I should be in an incurable or irreversible mental or physical condition with no reasonable expectation of recovery, it is my desire and intent that life-sustaining procedures and maintenance medical treatment be withheld and withdrawn. In such event, I direct all physicians and medical facilities in whose care I may be,

and my family, and all those concerned with my care, to refrain from and cease such life-sustaining procedures and maintenance medical treatment. These directions shall apply if (a) I am in a terminal condition, (b) I am permanently unconscious, or (c) I am conscious, but have irreversible brain damage and will never regain the ability to make decisions and express my wishes, or (d) two physicians conclude that there is no reasonable possibility of my being restored to a cognitive, sapient state. I hereby appoint and authorize my wife JENNIFER KEY, to act as my health care agent and attorney-in-fact to make and communicate all decisions about or relating to my receipt or refusal to accept medical treatment.

The ambiguity in this case is that it is not quite clear how terminal Mr. Key's condition is. He is unresponsive, but it is not clear that he has permanently lost consciousness. It does not look like he will ever be able to make decisions again, but this too is not definitively the case. So his living will can be interpreted in different ways, as is often the case. But in the final analysis, Mrs. Key must make a decision, as she is both her husband's legal agent and his authoritative family surrogate decision maker.

In this case Dr. Jacobs becomes convinced that, while he has every right to make recommendations to families, in the final analysis he was being too intrusive with his suggestion for dialysis. The ethics consultants were able to elicit Mrs. Key's discomfort with Dr. Jacobs's rather insistent attitude. Based on Mr. Key's advance directive, her own sense of what is best for him, and her daughter's position, the family as a whole achieves the desired consensus and determines that Mr. Key will be allowed to die comfortably, without dialysis.

It was important that Mrs. Key was the designated legal agent for Mr. Key because this allowed her to have a clear and unambiguous moral authority that Dr. Jacobs might otherwise not have fully respected, although her surrogate status as spouse would have been recognized in many states. The safest thing as a caregiver is to be a legally designated agent for health decisions via a durable power of attorney for health care. But do this early on while your loved one is still able to make such a designation!

Research Ethics

Several important passages are included below, taken from a definitive article in the *New England Journal of Medicine*:

> The legal approach to proxy decision making . . . relies on obtaining informed consent from a family member, identified on the basis of a hierarchy of family relationships widely thought to reflect closeness, such as spouse and then adult child. In many cases this hierarchy is also used to identify the person who is an ethically appropriate proxy for making decisions about participation in research. (Karlawish 2003, 1389)

> The core ethical challenge is to define the limits on the kinds of research risks that the proxy can accept on behalf of the noncompetent subject. (Karlawish 2003, 1390)

> A proxy should be allowed to enroll a person if the IRB finds that the research is potentially beneficial or presents minimal risks. . . . A common approach is to compare all risks of the research with all of the potential benefits for the subjects. The judgment that the risks are reasonable in relation to potential benefits . . . justifies the risks, even though they appear to be "greater than minimal." (Karlawish 2003, 1390)

In quick summary, in most research practice the individual with dementia who is able will be the primary source of informed consent but in the presence of their caregiver, who would generally want to cosign. If a person with dementia lacks capacity (a bit of a gray zone), then the decision rests entirely with the surrogate, based on what is in the loved one's best medical interests. In these situations, which are typical, the subject will still be present to the extent reasonable.

A proxy or surrogate does have to work within certain boundaries. The Association's statement from 2001 still stands (Alzheimer's 2001):

a. For minimal risk research all individuals should be allowed to enroll, even if there is no potential benefit to the individual. In the absence of an advance directive, proxy consent is acceptable.

b. For greater than minimal risk research *and* if there is a reasonable potential for benefit to the individual, the enrollment of all individuals with Alzheimer disease *is allowable based on proxy/surrogate consent.* The proxy's consent can be based on either a research specific advance directive *or* the proxy's judgment of the individual's best interests.

c. For greater than minimal risk research *and* if there is *no* reasonable potential for benefit to the individual only those individuals who (1) are capable of giving their own informed consent, or (2) have executed a research specific advance directive are allowed to participate. In either case, a proxy must be available to monitor the individual's involvement in the research.

If benefits are quite plausible and clear, the proxy or surrogate can make a best-interests decision even though the risks are slightly more than minimal. Surrogate consent should always be based on accurate facts about the risks and potential benefits of the clinical research or trial, rather than on understatement of risks or burdens and exaggerated claims of benefit. Participants in all research should be protected from significant pain or discomfort. It is the responsibility of all investigators and surrogates to monitor the well-being of participants.

INVESTIGATORS SHOULD

1. Rely for signed consent on the subject who has capacity but do so in the presence of caregiver/surrogate so they are fully aware and supportive and willing to cosign.

2. Clarify the identity of the family member to serve as a surrogate or the proxy decision maker legally designated in the event that the subject loses decisional capacity.

3. In gaining consent for the incapacitated subject, rely on the surrogate or legal proxy, but still involve the subject to whatever small extent is possible. While the subject's signature is no longer needed, it is nice to give him or her some opportunity to be involved.

7

"Is Grandma Still There?"

The Mystery of Continuing Self-Identity

As both a clinical ethicist and a pastoral caregiver, I listen attentively to caregivers who ask: Is Grandma still there beneath the breakdown in communication, the moments of emotional chaos, and the deep stillness? She is certainly still "there" as constituted by consciousness and by the sporadic expressions of continuing self-identity that appear to remain surprisingly intact beneath the surface of things. There is no compelling reason to think that she is absolutely "gone," although her capacity to communicate is heavily compromised by neurological atrophy. *Indeed, this book is based on the idea that at some profound level, deeply forgetful people are still present beneath confusion or silence, and they retain their worth and dignity.*

A number of important recent studies by leading researchers at top medical schools are beginning to confirm what caregivers have been saying all along about deeply forgetful people: yes, they are deeply forgetful, but no, they are not gone. Attention is now being given to anecdotes of "unexpected or paradoxical lucidity" in deeply forgetful people with long-standing dementia just days or weeks before death. Researchers from Yale, the University of Pennsylvania, the University of Virginia, and the University of Michigan write, "For the purposes of this article, paradoxical lucidity (PL) refers to an episode of unexpected, spontaneous, meaningful, and relevant communication or connectedness in a patient who is assumed to have permanently lost the capacity for coherent verbal or behavioral interaction due to a progressive and pathological dementing process" (Mashour et al. 2019, 1107). These researchers also cite various reports from physicians, nurses, and caregivers about PL on the last day of life, "the time shortly before the death of patients" (Mashour et al. 2019, 1107). In this context, the phenomenon is referred to as "terminal lucidity" or TL (Mashour et al. 2019, 1107). They offer no explanation of "the neurological underpinnings" of PL and TL, as it is very difficult to explain after so much neurological damage has occurred, although they suggest some possible mechanisms (Mashour et al. 2019, 1108). These neurological models are less than convincing because they do not explain how a fully lucid self-identity could possibly come back into view under such devastating conditions. In the first investigation of lucidity, 43 percent of these episodes occurred within the last day of life, 41 percent within two to seven days of death, and 10 percent within eight to thirty days of death (Nahm and Greyson 2009). In a brilliant 2020 article published by the American Psychological Association, researchers surveyed ten countries, including the United States, examining case reports of PL and TL. In 80 percent of 124 detailed reports of patients with dementia, caregivers reported "complete remission with return of memory, orientation, and responsive verbal ability" as reported by direct observers (Batthyany and Greyson 2020, 1).

Having seen several episodes of terminal lucidity myself, I am comfortable with these studies, which are now appearing in the leading scientific journals, such as *Alzheimer's & Dementia* and *Psychology of Consciousness: Theory, Research, and Practice.* With old Grandma

Post I always felt intuitively that she was there behind the silence. One of the nicest things about the Music and Memory movement is that when deeply forgetful people who have been "out of it" for long periods hear music that is deeply learned and meaningful to them from earlier in life, the majority will quicken in their bodily rhythmic expressions and begin to chime in with a little singing, after which for a brief few minutes they may even be capable of conversation, indicating that now they can remember who they are. The stirring video documentary on this phenomenon, *Alive Inside: A Story of Music and Memory* (2014), captures social worker Dan Cohen demonstrating the immensely successful use of this particular brief form of music therapy in bringing people with Alzheimer's "back into who they are."

I am not suggesting that such musically induced returns to fleeting lucidity prove the existence of an immortal soul. It is possible that despite neurological devastation there are still some remnants of selfhood under the surface of things that arise to expression with the right stimulus. Yet this is hard to explain because the intactness of personhood and self-identity is so complete.

"Paradoxical" or "Terminal" Lucidity

In addition to working with Music and Memory interventions along with medical students, I have personally witnessed three cases of perfect terminal lucidity in people with Alzheimer's who were within hours of death, and I have been told about several dozen others, some of whom I described in chapter two. The term "terminal lucidity" (also know as "paradoxical lucidity") was first used in 2009 by German biologist Michael Nahm in his article in *The Journal of Near-Death Studies*. Nahm, a leader in the study of consciousness, pointed out that accounts of cognitively impaired people becoming lucid as their death approaches have a long history but lacked a formal name. He defined terminal lucidity as follows: "The (re-)emergence of normal or unusually enhanced mental abilities in dull, unconscious, or mentally ill patients shortly before death" (Nahm 2009).

Nahm and University of Virginia psychiatrist Bruce Greyson teamed up that same year in their article "Terminal Lucidity in Patients with Chronic Schizophrenia and Dementia," which appeared in the prestigious *Journal of Nervous and Mental Disease* (Nahm and Greyson 2009). Then, with two additional authors, they published "Terminal Lucidity: A Review and a Case Collection," in *Archives of Gerontology and Geriatrics* (Nahm et al. 2012), in which they trace reports of terminal lucidity in medical literature for over 250 years. In these cases, 84 percent occurred within a week of death; 43 percent occurred on the final day of life. They cite a study in which 70 percent of caregivers in a British nursing home said that they had personally observed people with dementia becoming lucid shortly before their deaths, although it must immediately be stated that only ten people worked there. In one case a ninety-two-year-old woman with advanced Alzheimer's who had not recognized her family members in years or communicated verbally suddenly on the day of her death recalled their names and had a bright conversation.

In terminal lucidity we have a real medical mystery that seems difficult to explain at this time. Somehow the essence of the self that was otherwise buried in brain atrophy rises into the foreground to be heard from again as if fully intact. Harvard neurologist Rudy Tanzi, intrigued by this occurrence, has produced a number of impressive videos about consciousness, terminal lucidity, and dementia that are readily available on the internet.

I am not trying to be scientifically persuasive in this chapter, but I draw on what science is available to leave the door slightly open for mystery. Mystery is a term Roman Catholic neurologist Joseph M. Foley often invoked to explain such phenomena. I also acknowledge several conversations at the University of Chicago with Nobel Laureate Sir John Eccles (1903-1997), who for all his work on the basic physiology of brain synapses, held firmly that mind is more than brain and even a separate substance.

On Spirituality

I write only for caregivers, so many of whom believe in a soul that materialism rejects. *Why is this question of soul so relevant for caregivers?* In the presence of Grandma Post, even as she became more forgetful, it never once occurred to me that her life was of any less value than my own or than anyone else's. We cannot claim with any certainty that these three aspects of a human being—consciousness, enduring essence, and continuing selfhood—are absent. This mystery may be beyond the explanatory grasp of current neuroscience. At least this is what the great ancient religions suggest, especially the Hindu tradition, but including all traditions that do not take a strictly materialist perspective regarding mind and person. It is possible that our minds and memories are not fully explicable in terms of brain cells and tissue alone, physical substances that inevitably deteriorate with aging. People become deeply forgetful and senile, but no spiritual (nonmaterialist) thinkers have suggested that they are not still one with the eternal. As Ralph Waldo Emerson posited, we are all a small drop of an oceanic mind or oversoul even when we are no longer masters of intellect, memory, and will.

Hindus greet one another with "Namaste," meaning roughly: "I honor the place in you that is the same in me. I honor the place in you where the whole universe resides. I honor the place in you of love, of light, of peace and of truth. I honor the place in you that is the same in me." As human beings and as caregivers, we respect a deeply forgetful person as still, to quote a Hindu sage, "a god among gods." Dismiss all thoughts of the inferiority of the person before you and give yourself no air of arrogance. But never think that deeply forgetful people are not your equals, and trust in their inner light rather than in reason.

Metaphysics aside—and I do not wish to claim that a purely materialistic interpretation of paradoxical or terminal lucidity will not suffice as we learn more about consciousness—I saw Grandma Post as "still there," as "alive inside," and therefore as someone with whom I could develop empathy and build bridges of connectivity.

No doubt my use of the term "deeply forgetful" is suggestive of continuing self-identity, and perhaps it has some quasi-mystical overtones, but it certainly suggests an appreciation for mystery and for a view of the human essence that is at least open to some sort of "soulishness," which is of course the view of the billions of people who hold to the nonmaterialist view of the inner human being. When these many caregivers ensconced in their spiritual traditions affirm something literally eternal in a loved one, we need to at least be culturally sensitive and show respect. It is from an affirmation of soul that their right attitudes will follow, and that their love is expressed.

Maybe that deeply forgetful person is more in inward harmony with the infinite than we have ever known as we rush around from place to place trapped in the demands of chronological time and life's countless pressures. Think about the value that every civilization has placed on the human soul in one way or another, and recommended that we love our neighbor as ourselves, making their well-being and security as meaningful to us as our own.

A Trip to Bangalore

This chapter may be considered a bit "outside the box" by the materialist scientific researchers with whom I sometimes work, but I am not writing to please them. I write exclusively in response to the voices of caregivers as I have known them for decades all over North America, for the vast majority of whom dementia raises perennial metaphysical questions about human nature and spirituality. To ignore spirituality would be to ignore their voices.

But nevertheless, I did not gather up my determination to write this chapter until I arrived at the Indian National Institute for Advanced Studies in Bangalore, surrounded by great Hindu philosophers and leading Indian neuroscientists. All the people I met there were in sync with my ideas and took them seriously. Nothing is proven in this chapter, although perhaps open-mindedness is made more plausible. At any rate, it is a chapter written for everyday folks, many of whom hold to deeply spiritual assumptions.

"Is Grandma still there?" This is the big metaphysical question that most caregivers ask when it comes to their loved ones with dementia. I asked it as a young man caring for my grandmother on visits to the nursing home. It is a desperate question driven by the need to find spiritual and moral meaning in many difficult endeavors. Time and again, over thirty years of consulting with families, I have been asked just this question. I have encountered many caregivers who view the syndrome of dementia in its various forms (including Alzheimer's disease) as a breakdown in the capacity of the brain to connect with a still complete and forever intact biographical selfhood. Caregivers' spiritual-metaphysical assumption is not that the hints at continuing self-identity are mere remnants of a mostly "gone" self as located in residual brain tissue. Rather, they view the brain more like a computer that can no longer retrieve memories from cloud storage, although those memories remain perfectly intact in an unseen mystery of immortality. One caregiver said to me, "Stephen, it was St. Paul in Romans 8:39 who wrote that absolutely nothing can separate us from the love of God, and that includes Alzheimer's for sure." I did not know quite how to respond, but I would never deride such a commonly held view, although it falls outside of the range of science. This book is for caregivers, as I have said.

The materialist may deem the idea of any nonmaterial memory substrate, however defined, as nonsensical. But so many caregivers nevertheless assert, "We know Grandma is still fully there, underneath the chaos and the silence, with an eternal soul that is slowly returning to the arms of the Supreme."

Fifteen Focus Groups

In a series of fifteen focus groups on spirituality with deeply forgetful individuals and their families, I was struck by comments from several people who stated that while they had very little memory left, they did not miss their memories because now they were living mostly in the present—so the past did not matter. As one man said, "I may not remember anything much, but I have my rosary and I am just fine praying." His wife said that he prays more now than ever, although he always prayed occasionally, and that even if he could remember more she was not sure he wanted to because living in the present is more than enough to live fully. I referred to these groups as "Circles of Spiritual Trust," which the participants all appreciated since it is less technical sounding and more meaningful than "focus groups."

I learned in the Circles that deeply forgetful people are in a new stage of life in which the past and the future fade away, and they experience full consciousness in the now. People spend most of their years adjusting to the physical material world around them and all of its stressful demands. These chronological pressures and related productivity demands make it hard for them to pause and find time for some other way of being—a spiritual way. They are here exploring consciousness in the now, and through small focus groups and good facilitation they can connect in the present with their inner being and with others in ways that are actually refreshing. In a Circle of Spiritual Trust they are treated with kindness, respect, acceptance, and gratitude.

This level of spiritual appreciation for deeply forgetful people requires family members and caregivers to transcend worry about capacities and memories that seem lost. Emphatically, if someone forgot the name of a loved one in a Circle it was nothing to be concerned about, and everyone assumed that the connective presence was still there. No one felt hurt or despaired when a name was forgotten. The trust was deep enough so that names meant little. Sometimes I have seen family members put far too much emphasis on the fact that "the other day Grandma forgot my name" and then launch into some intense emotional reaction as though Grandma was gone. We all forget names all the time, but a deeply forgetful person will remember names better under the right circumstances and after a refreshing sleep. People can forget many names often and still be fully present.

An appreciation for the spirit of deep forgetfulness does not mean that we should not keep trying to reconnect deeply forgetful people with the things that they can still do and enjoy through art, poetry, nature, creativity, personalized music, and the like. However, it is a good idea to balance our desire to support them in what they can still do with simply appreciating the fullness of their consciousness in the moment. Let us assume that deeply forgetful people are perhaps in closer touch with the spiritual essence of their existence than most of us are as we rush around pursuing our ego goals and seeking rational linear truth. It might be good for all of us to put aside those ego goals and discover a form of truth that is not intellectual but rather a matter of being aware of the moment and all that goes on within it.

Yes indeed, there is a certain blessing in forgetting about self and in enjoying the truth of the now. I have always told caregivers that while there are all kinds of spiritual books about living in the now and practices to transcend time, when they are in the presence of a deeply forgetful person there is no choice but to live mostly in the now, although again, it is good to notice and encourage the whispers and expressions of continuing selfhood beneath the surface.

To certain religious believers, it is as though deeply forgetful people are ahead of the game in the process of a gradual passing from this world, for they have already taken one large step away from this earth and have one foot in a world of spirit. They are slowly moving away from the world, and in this process they are in a phase of life that frees them from attachments and brings them closer to a spiritual essence. Of course, to take this seriously one has to think that an eternal soul is still there underneath all the chaos of dementia, seeking peace.

Over the years, I have often worked with faith communities to teach them how to form small Circles of Spiritual Trust (of no more than eight people) for deeply forgetful people and their caregivers. Not only does the Circle diminish stress for all involved, but it frees everyone. It is best to begin with a minute of silence, a well-known hymn, and a brief prayer, and then just see what follows. Often, deeply forgetful people are more spiritual than we could have imagined, even if they are just sitting quietly in the moment with a look of tranquil joy.

A Speculative Model of Continuing Selfhood

Nobody really knows what memory is, physically or metaphysically, and so it remains a mystery. I am not trying to prove anything scientifically, but for all the thousands of family members who have asked me about memory over the decades, I must address the question in an open-minded way.

In the 1920s neuroscientist Wilder Penfield offered evidence that specific memories are located in specific areas of the brain in the form of "engrams" or memory traces. But in the 1940s neuropsychologist Karl Lashley, after decades of research on the brains of rats, concluded that memories are not found in specific brain locations but are instead distributed "globally" throughout the brain as a whole. The idea that memory is distributed globally over a neural network—an idea taken up later by Donald Hebbs—in some synaptic associations is indeed interesting, but also unproven and highly questionable. This fact drove one of Lashley's students, neuropsychologist Karl Pribram of Yale, to develop the idea that the brain is in some mysterious way holographic, meaning that all memory, including the whole of a life, is contained in each and every brain location. While this idea is quite interesting, the model lacks any empirical support. It may be proven true one day, and some have tried to defend it articulately (Talbot 2011).

The narrative memories that constitute self-identity do have infinite "megabytes" of information, and even the smallest microchips lack the capacity to store this infinity. It is said that small computers can hold a great amount of memory, so by analogy we look within the brain to unlock this boundlessness. But at a certain point, this sort of model breaks down logically, because it is easier to view the brain not as a finite cupboard for infinite vastness, but rather as a transmission device. To use television as an analogy, TV shows are not inside the TV but outside of it. The infinite cannot be contained in the finite, or so the argument would go.

Given how little we know, let us be respectfully open-minded with those caregivers who affirm the eternal essence of self-identity. It is possible that the brain is an uploading and downloading device that has space for habituations such as those a rat develops in learning a maze, but not for the infinity of our life histories and related endless imaginings. Of course, this model opens the door for higher inspiration, synchronicity, premonitions, and the like. But my focus is merely memory here.

It may be true that all the hints at continuing self-identity in deeply forgetful people are the last disintegrating remnants of a person's autobiographical self as located in an entirely "local" and deteriorating brain. Yes, perhaps the large number of synaptic connections will someday explain all things. And it is true that no one has proven the reality of a nonmaterial soul that exists in an unseen dimension of reality. Still, logic suggests that a fathomless sea of infinite richness and textual detail is too much to engrave in a small mass of chemicals, cells, synapses, and tissue. Contrary to even the most "nonreductive" of the physicalists, we need not give up on our eternal souls just yet, although some theologians have given up on theirs (Brown, Murphy, and Malony 1998).

Some very thoughtful philosophers and scientists assert the eternal soul. The list is a long one and includes, for example, Plato, the author of Genesis, the author of The Gospel of John, St. Paul, Buddha, Mohammed, Jesus Christ, Meister Eckhart, T. S. Eliot, C. S. Lewis, J. R. R. Tolkien, Ralph Waldo Emerson, David Bohm, William James, C. G. Jung, Ken Wilber, Huston Smith, Aldous Huxley, Larry Dossey, Seyyed Hossein Nasr, Sir John Templeton, and Joseph Campbell.

One of the most respected philosophers of our time, Thomas Nagel, in his book *Mind and Cosmos: Why the Materialist Neo-Darwinian Conception of Nature Is Almost Certainly False,* comments that his doubts about materialism will strike most people as "outrageous" because they have been "browbeaten" to believe in a mindless universe (Nagel 2013, 7). But Nagel takes a view very different from materialism—"one that makes mind central, rather than a side effect" of the material (Nagel 2013, 15).

The Continuing Mystery of Autobiographical Memory

The Muslim philosopher Avicenna, along with Augustine in his famous *Confessions*, waxed eloquent about how in memory we can envision and hear the entire universe and everything we have encountered in life. The great Hindu sages asserted the same thing, and therefore held that memory is an aspect of consciousness or mind that is primary in itself, underived from matter. What we can call up and envision from memory with eyes closed is unlimited in detail and scope, although the brain retrieval of information is complex, as well as potentially inaccurate at times (Brady et al. 2008).

The French theophilosopher Henri Bergson, in his classic 1896 work *Matter and Memory: An Essay on the Relation of Body and Spirit* (1994), described aspects of image remembrance and personal narrative as profoundly spiritual in nature. In Bergson's view the brain has a retrieval function, but brain injuries then do not erase that which they retrieve. Bergson acknowledged that the brain is the locus of engrained habituated memories, as we find in many nonhuman animals as well as humans, but not of "image remembrance" of the past, or "pure" memory, which is of a contemplative and nonmaterial nature. Bergson concluded, "The idea that the body preserves memories in the mechanical form of cerebral deposits, that the loss or decrease of memory consists in their more or less complete destruction, whereas the heightening of memory and hallucination consists in an excess of their activity, is not, then, borne out by either reasoning or by the facts" (Bergson 1994, 176). He asserts that memory is "absolutely independent of matter" (Bergson 1994, 177). For Bergson, it seems that the brain is more an organ of perception and habituation than of storage. The cupboard of autobiographical memory lies elsewhere.

A line of contrarian neuroscience today asserts that we need a paradigm shift in our thinking about memory. In 1993, Simon Y. Berkovich of George Washington University presented a speculative model of the brain as the local computer terminal connecting to some larger informational system. Fifteen years later, writing in the highly regarded *Proceedings of the National Academy of Sciences*, T. F. Brady and team showed just how massive visual memory is, and concluded that it seems to "pose a challenge to neural models of memory storage and retrieval, which must be able to account for such a large and detailed storage capacity" (Brady et al. 2008, 14325). This is no trivial challenge to the reigning paradigm.

In the late 1970s the renowned British pediatric neurologist John Lorber famously reported that some perfectly intelligent adults with fine memories had no more than 5 percent of normal brain tissue after having been cured as children of hydrocephaly (water on the brain). Roger Lewin's 1980 article entitled "Is Your Brain Really Necessary?," which appeared in *Science*, dismissed Lorber's research as unscientific and "overdramatic." While initially disbelieved, Lorber's observations, based on brain scans, have been confirmed by a team of French neurologists (Feuillet, Dufour, and Pelletier 2007).

Bringing this quarrel up to date, Donald R. Forsdyke (2015) in his article "Wittengenstein's Certainty Is Uncertain: Brain Scans of Cured Hydrocephalics Challenge Cherished Assumptions," appearing in *Bio-*

logical Theory, urges the open-mindedness that Lorber's work seems to press upon us. Forsdyke, a distinguished researcher at Queen's University in Ontario, has studied microcephalic cases where intelligence as well as long-term memory are normal. He reports that information content and memory do not correlate with head size, and he cites Fusi and Abbott (2007), with their calls for a radical remodeling of memory. Because brain size does not scale with information quantity, Forsdyke gives us three hypotheses to work with:

1. The "standard model" posits that long-term memory is held in the brain in some chemical or physical form.
2. Long-term memory is held in the brain by "some extremely minute, subatomic form, as yet unknown to biochemists and physiologists" but akin to computers storing large amounts of information in progressively smaller spaces.
3. "Information relating to long-term memory is held outside the brain. Since most nonneural tissues and organs appear unsuited to the task, this extrapolates to long-term memory being *outside* the body—extracorporeal! Amazingly, this startling alternative has been on the table for at least two decades." (Forsdyke 2015, 339)

It is hard for scientists raised under the ideology of materialism to imagine this third alternative. But for most religious people in all the great spiritual traditions, mind (which also goes by ultimate reality, Platonic *nous*, supreme being, eternal consciousness, infinite mind, pure unlimited love, ground of being, God, and so on) precedes and sustains mere matter. It is certain that bone marrow creates blood cells, but there is no fully convincing evidence that neural tissue produces mind, conscious awareness, biographical memory, and the like.

This all remains a mystery and we must keep abreast of the new science and biological models. But perhaps there is something to the ancient idea of mind before matter, as examined in the edited volume *Beyond Physicalism: Toward Reconciliation of Science and Spirituality*, which contains two chapters on a "cloud storage" model of memory (Kelly, Crabtree, and Marshall 2015). This volume was recommended to me by the distinguished psychiatrist Bruce Greyson of the University of Virginia, who has contributed immensely to the study of paradoxical and terminal lucidity.

Consciousness as the Ground of Personhood and Dignity

Consciousness is everything going on within a mind in the moment and includes connectedness with others and with the outside world. Emotional states such as awe and kindness, relational presence, and environmental awareness are all constitutive of consciousness. One does not need a strong connection with time or with logical and intellectual skill sets to be fully conscious. Consciousness is deeper than reason, and it is the ground of being insofar as we participate in some form of universal mind that connects us in mysterious ways through dreams and intuitions.

The leading British philosopher-psychiatrist Dr. Julian C. Hughes has written an article entitled "Beyond Hypercognitivism: A Philosophical Basis for Good Quality Palliative Care in Dementia." He begins as follows:

> When Stephen Post introduced, in 1995, the term "hypercognitive" he had in view "a persistent bias against the deeply forgetful that is especially pronounced in modern philosophical accounts of the 'person'." He has stated that when the capacity to seek meaning in the midst of decline gives way to more advanced dementia . . . then the experience of the person must be understood in relational and affective terms rather than in narrowly cognitive ones. (Hughes 2006, 18)

Hughes then proceeds to develop the notion of "human conscious-ness," in contrast to "self-consciousness." Western philosophers have followed the Oxford Enlightenment thinker John Locke in emphasiz-ing "self-consciousness" as the basis of being a "person," for a person is a being able to "consider itself as self" (Hughes 2006, 19). Memory plays the key role in self-consciousness then, for without it "the glue that holds together the self is gone" (Hughes 2006, 19). Hughes rejects this influential Lockean view of "personhood" as "self-consciousness" and replaces it with the broader "human consciousness" that "calls to mind everything that might be involved in human mental life" (Hughes 2006, 19). He argues that "in other words, the notion of hu-man consciousness brings in Post's emotional, relational, and aes-thetic aspects of personhood" (Hughes 2006, 19).

Human Consciousness and Post-Materialism

Perhaps unlike Hughes—although I may be wrong—I think of "hu-man consciousness" in terms of a nonmaterial soul. Good careful science should never be interfered with. But whether we interpret findings in a materialist or a post-materialist metaphysical model is a matter where we should welcome diversity. One hundred sci-entists from a variety of fields convened at the Canyon Ranch in Tucson, Arizona, from February 7 through 9, 2014, to discuss the emergence of a post-materialist paradigm for science, spirituality, and society. This group produced *The Manifesto for a Post-Materialist Sci-ence* (http://opensciences.org/about/manifesto-for-a-post-materialist-science). The manifesto challenges the nineteenth-century assump-tion, now turned into dogma and known as "scientific materialism," and in particular the belief that "mind is nothing but the physical ac-tivity of the brain, and that our thoughts cannot have any effect upon our brains and bodies, our actions, and the physical world." These experts argue that we need a new and non-dogmatic science that follows the methods of the best science but does not presume materialist explanations.

It is for many religious people very difficult to affirm the human dignity and moral status of the deeply forgetful unless we place some faith in the idea that every human being has within a drop of the infinite cloud or some sort of supreme being. The famous materialist philosopher Bertrand Russell was at least able to acknowledge that if materialism is true, if all we are is an admixture of chemicals and cells, then the sum total of the meaning of a human life is no greater than bacterial "pond scum."

But let us put these metaphysical questions aside and accept for the moment the comfortable materialist's assumption that human beings have no eternal soul or selfhood. Let us assert, however, that even on the materialist paradigm, continuity of self-identity in the deeply forgetful is the residual or remnant norm, and that this remnant does afford them due respect.

Hope in Deep Self-Identity

I define hope in the experience of caregivers as "openness to surprises," at least in the context of dementia. In other contexts hope might be defined very differently—for example in terms of the pursuit of clearly envisioned goals. My student, in a vignette repeated from chapter two, chose to focus his essay on his mother's interaction with her father just before his death:

> *It was in his last moments that my mother seemed to be rewarded for all her hard work. My grandfather looked at my mother and spoke to her with complete lucidity for the first time in a year. He talked about the old times when he used to walk her to school. Then he talked about me and told her to make sure I kept working hard in school. And the last*

thing he said was how proud he was of her and that he loved her. The
next morning he was gone.

Again, hope is being open to surprises such as my student describes.

Over the years of witnessing many cases of sudden insight, I ask: Where does such lucidity come from? Yes, it could be some remnant of a neurologically grounded memory if personal identity and biographical memory actually exist in matter, which from the perspective of a purely megabyte analysis can be and is being questioned. But it could also be a sign that underneath the neurological deterioration a whole self continues on. Given the current state of brain science, we must all be agnostic. We simply do not know. Moments of lucidity are the norm among the deeply forgetful, rather than the exception, especially early in the morning after a good night's rest. Do they point toward remnants of autobiographical narrative in a devastated brain, or to something fully intact housed in "cloud storage" but now more difficult to access?

Whatever the answer, ethically we need to respect cultures and families where the soul is more than neurology and has an eternal quality, even if we happen not to believe in such ideas. A great many people still do.

A Pastoral Conclusion

One need not be a metaphysical nonmaterialist who believes in an eternal soul to observe that hypercognitive values discriminate badly against the deeply forgetful, who have other aspects of the self that are as important as cognition, and even more so, including these aspects: symbolic, creative, emotional, relational, somatic, musical, rhythmic, aesthetic, olfactory, spiritual, and tactile.

I am an ethicist-pastor to deeply forgetful people and their families. Whether you believe in an eternal soul or you believe that mind and memory are all merely in the brain tissue, we can agree on this: when it comes to the deeply forgetful love is the question, love is the answer, and love is the way—even in the hard times when caring feels overwhelming and perhaps for the moment even a bit meaningless, although it is always meaningful. It is all about the power of love, not about the love of hypercognitive power. After all, we can hopefully acknowledge that in an era of heightened sensitivity to the equal moral status of people with physical and cognitive disabilities, we should not dismiss the consciousness and awareness of an individual with dementia as somehow less significant than that of someone who is more lucid of mind.

"Is Grandma still there?" I always affirm caregivers who believe in the eternal soul of a loved one with a simple reply: "You could be right, but I do not know." I stay open-minded and respectful of their beliefs, and it is in this sense that I offer this chapter to them.

An Epilogue

North Wind

The following narrative was written by a thoughtful theologian in response to the preceding chapters. Because his parents are still alive, he preferred to leave the authorship anonymous.

The quiet sounds of running water and conversation drift in from the kitchen, punctuated by the occasional clacking of dirty dinner plates. I cannot make out the words, but no doubt Mom is holding forth on the difficulty of life in general, while my wife nods respectfully and listens. My children and my father are elsewhere in the house, the home my parents purchased just months ago. For years we had prodded them to move closer to us. Your health isn't what it used to be, we said, and *we* can't move closer to you. "Can't"—such a convenient, ambiguous word, as if some universal law stood in the way. We would have had to give up our careers, sever the children from their schools, their friends. Of course, we can't, we couldn't. But I also knew that there was another side: my parents had lived in the same area where I grew up for the entirety of their life together. These roots went deep, and they did not yield easily. There is no easy calculus for such sacrifices.

Together, we inspected a variety of houses, at first no more than a formal exercise in imagining new possibilities. This one? Each house turned out to be unsuitable in its own way: too old, too dark, too close to the freeway. Had it been my grandmother, the verdict might have been too unlucky. Between visits, however, it seemed that fate itself conspired with circumstance to loosen the ties that bound them to home. The friends they had known for decades began, one by one, to forsake this life, and those who were left behind were forced to rethink their own mortality. It was then that the right house revealed itself, at a not too unreasonable price—clean and recently built, suggesting fresh beginnings.

Door to door, we are only a few miles away, as compared to the hundreds that separated us for twenty years. Now, with teenagers at home and aging parents nearby, we have entered what some call the "sandwich" generation. I dislike the metaphor. But if there is any truth to it, then my wife is the meat, the sustenance. I am . . . mustard, perhaps, or some other condiment, added for character and flavor. Between the two of us, she is the more responsibly aware, anticipating and filling needs. I wait to be told what to do and consider myself praiseworthy for having meticulously followed the directions I have been given.

Something inside me feels out of sync, like waking up in a strange place and wondering if I'm dreaming. In hindsight, I realize that part of me has been caught unawares; I had not expected the years to slip away like this. When was it, exactly, that my parents became old? And the other side, just as uncertain: when did I stop being young?

I am alone in the living room, setting up the table for our weekly game of mah-jongg, or "M.J." as my parents call it. The tiles clatter insistently as I shuffle them back and forth across the tabletop, then stack them into walls.

I have done this ever since I was a child, setting up the game when my parents' friends would come to gamble the evening away. To be an enduring part of that circle, one apparently had to meet at least three out of four requirements, one cultural, the other three a matter of avocation. Being Chinese was a must. Beyond that, a fondness for bowling, poker, and mah-jongg were the required assets, not necessarily in that order. My siblings and I were taught the first two early on, but we were never initiated into the latter, with its mysteriously colorful markings and glyphs. It's like gin rummy, we were told. But we knew how to play rummy, and this was different. Maybe my parents thought the game too complicated for us to understand, or maybe we were more interested in being American than Chinese. Maybe both; I don't know.

But I knew how to set up the table. My mother, being handier than my father, had made a custom tabletop just for the game. She covered it with green Naugahyde and sized it to fit snugly over a card table that had been given to them as a wedding present. It was my job to make sure that all was ready for the game. I would greet the guests as they arrived, addressing them as "Uncle" and "Auntie," though they bore no relation to me, and then retire to my room. I can remember lying in the dark, listening to the distant sound of tiles being shuffled for the next hand, like the sound of a hard rain slapping against the patio. Countless nights, I would slide into sleep on that familiar clatter.

Now, decades later, I am once again in my parents' living room, setting up. It's a new home, but the same table. The Naugahyde has lost most of its faux-leather smell, and the card table beneath wobbles unsteadily on spindly legs, half a century old. We could buy another table, and I could easily make a new top for it. But I would never dream of suggesting such a thing. Neither would anyone else.

The difference is that I have learned to play. So has my wife, who is not Chinese. And so have my children, who are at best half Chinese—though I wonder from time to time if they have any truly Asian blood in them at all. So we sit one evening a week, after the dinnertime detritus has been cleared away: three generations around a table, playing a game that seems as ancient as the Chinese culture itself.

We begin with the east wind. I sit across from my father, who is now well into his eighties. He is as animated and happy as I ever see him, a more alert version of himself than the one who so frequently sits entranced by cable TV. His hands move quickly and surely when snapping tiles together in formation; he rolls the dice with a practiced flick. Dad loves this game. He is disappointed when we don't play, even if he doesn't say anything about it.

I arrange my tiles into suits, bemoaning my usual poor luck as if it were my part in the family script. I glance across the table at Dad, who is scowling at his own hand. There's something more than just the game, though, reflected in his face. With each year that passes, he's looking more and more like his mother.

We called her Yin-Yin, "Grandma" in her dialect. She spoke little English, and I never learned to speak Chinese. Nor did I see her often. Visiting the grandparents was a duty that children and grandchildren accepted without question. Affection, if it existed, seemed irrelevant. My relationship to Yin-Yin was simple. I would smile and gingerly offer a peck on her softly sagging cheek, aware of the fusty smell of her shawl. She offered glasses of cold milk, and on special occasions, the traditional red envelope of lucky money. My memories of her are from when she lived with one of my uncles and his family. In her waning years, though, she was under the care of my father's only sister, who shouldered the greatest part of her mother's mental erosion after Grandfather died.

The deterioration lasted nearly a decade, sliding inexorably from absentmindedness to the inability to recognize her own family, the very children she had birthed. My aunt would come home from shopping, and Yin-Yin would lock her out of the house, thinking her to be an intruder. My aunt had to plead to be admitted to her own home. Nor was it necessarily a happy occasion when Yin-Yin did recognize one of her children. Number three uncle went to pay his respects and was rewarded with torrential invective about the worthless son that was no better than dead to her. He patiently withstood the onslaught as best he could, then left unceremoniously.

What few traditions our rather disconnected family observed were eventually washed away in the tide that took my grandmother's memory. It had been the custom to honor the grandparents with a banquet on their birthdays. Several tables were reserved at one of the family's favorite Chinese eateries, and her five children gathered to take her to dinner. She was docile and cooperative and ate well; her physical strength had not suffered the same decline. But when the time came to leave, she would not get in the car. My father and his siblings pleaded and struggled with her, growing more embarrassed and angry at the public spectacle they were enacting on the sidewalk in front of the crowded restaurant. Convinced that she was being kidnapped by strangers, she fought furiously, screaming and cursing in Cantonese. I don't know how they actually got her home that evening. To my knowledge, there was no banquet the following year.

My mother tells me that she volunteered to care for her mother-in-law for a short while, so that my aunt could have some much-deserved respite. Yin-Yin came to live with my parents for a mere ten days, which Mom describes as being ten of the longest days of her life. Much of Yin-Yin's behavior was innocuous enough. She refused to change her clothes, even for bed, and slept curled up on top of the covers. But she couldn't be left alone. One afternoon, unable to remember where the bathroom was, she bolted out the door and attempted to relieve herself in the front yard. When she heard my parents shouting and running, she too ran, her undergarments still pulling at her ankles.

Again, though, she ate reasonably well, until the last day, when my aunt was scheduled to retrieve her. Mom cooked a good Chinese meal and set it in front of her, but Yin-Yin refused to eat. Mom and Dad tried to ask her why, but she remained mute and anxiously shook her head. It was not until my aunt arrived and scolded her that the reason was revealed. She couldn't eat the food, she said, because she didn't have any money, and couldn't pay these people, whoever they were.

The stories of my grandmother's decline into dementia continue to haunt the family, long after her departure. My mother paints vivid word pictures of Yin-Yin's final days in a nursing home, sitting in a chair for hours, oblivious to her surroundings, chuckling occasionally to some private joke. Whole days would be spent staring at her hands as they clutched and unclutched around the tatters of an old shawl, hers or somebody else's—nobody knew. These tales and images have become a benchmark of sorts, against which the functioning of my father's generation is silently but surely measured. Simple acts of forgetfulness take on the more exalted status of warning signs, dark harbingers of the approaching storm. Nor have I, at one generation further removed, been immune to these self-fulfilling prophecies. At the office, I miss an appointment, or forget promises made. Driving, I distractedly run a stop sign. Rather than shrug them off as normal lapses, I wonder instead if the plot line of mental absence is indelibly written into the generations. A few short decades from now, will I be too dangerous to be allowed on the streets? And how will I respond when my children come to separate me from my driver's license?

These days, Mom worries that Dad is more and more following in his mother's path. He is already past the age that she was when she began her slide. He wears a pacemaker as his father before him had. It was Grandfather's failed pacemaker that killed him, in hindsight a merciful death. Dad almost died a few years back, when his heart raced out of control and he collapsed in the bowling alley. Then, Mom was panicked because she wasn't ready. She is now. Given the choice, a heart attack in the bowling alley seems infinitely preferable to watching him suffer his mother's fate. Mom reads it daily in the blank expressions he returns to her questions, or his increasing irascibility. She worries, too, that she herself is more forgetful than she used to be, and wonders where it all must lead. Death, if it visits swiftly and without undue shame, is not unwelcome in this house.

For the moment, though, I watch as Dad pounces on the tile he needs to win. The east wind round is finished. We pay his winnings in pink and green chips, and he chatters triumphantly about how hard it was to put together that particular hand. He would tell you that he doesn't play the game as well as he once did, that he sometimes forgets what he is doing, or misses a play for want of better concentration. From my vantage point as a mere novitiate, though, I admire how much easier the game is for my parents than for me.

Tonight, he retires early from the game. The rest of us are weary as well, each from a long day of school or work. We hardly ever seem to get all the way around the compass points to the north wind, a full game. So, we are finished for the evening. The card table is returned to its proper place, and the tiles are neatly arranged in their leather case, safe in the cupboard. We bid my parents good night and thank Mom for a lovely dinner. Next week, same time? Of course.

Later, I am lying in bed awaiting sleep. The kids have reluctantly extinguished the lights in their rooms, and my wife is already breathing deeply and evenly at my side. Sighing, I roll over on my side, stare into the darkness, and wonder. What will happen when I have reached my eighties, should the unsearchable God permit it to be so? I realize that to some extent, as I am learning anew the role of the dutiful son, I am performing for my own children. See, kids, this is what to do when your parents get old; this is what is right.

But I want neither to be a mere player, nor for my children to act merely out of compulsion. Visit me, care for me, talk to me, because you want to, not because you have to, not because you have to check me off on your list of morally right things to do. I sometimes feel divided between the ideals of duty and affection, between love expressed as filial piety and love experienced as a desire to care for those who loved me and gave me life. My parents want me to want them, and they are sensitive to the subtle or clumsy social cues that say, no, not tonight, we're too busy for you.

Honor your father and mother, the commandment says, carved in stone by the finger of God, yet perhaps less permanently inscribed on the fleshly tablet of my own heart. I love my parents. I do not think of them as a burden; they are my parents. But unlike the God who commands that we love him and each other, my affections are not unalloyed. When will my loyalty to my parents be overcome by loyalty to myself, my freedom, my sovereignty in matters of time and choice? As a family, we have not yet faced the deepest challenges; we have only felt the fringes of the cloak of forgetfulness that may eventually cover my father's shoulders. We do not know what the future may bring, good or ill. And yet in the recesses of my imagination, I feel the tingle of apprehension. In truth, I am afraid: afraid for him, afraid for my mother. For my wife, and for my children. I am afraid for me. But over the rattling of uncertainty, I still hear the persistent whisper of duty, the command that lingers and prods.

To a God who loved the universe into being, is duty enough? It seems a poor substitute for affectionate devotion. The parable of the prodigal son weighs on me, in which the coldly dutiful elder brother seems wooden and surly in contrast to the unabashed and joyful love of the father. Such exuberance is foreign to me. But perhaps, too, I have lived too long in a world and a culture where love is defined as spontaneous emotion, and duty is the unwanted taskmaster. I don't know if my forebears would have understood this. Did my aunt wonder about these things as she cared for her mother all those long, wearisome years? Ah, yes, those Americans, always so concerned about their feelings.

The whisperings will not go away. In matters of devotion, duty will be my tutor, an obedience that reshapes both my affections and my fears. Its discipline will become less demanding when I allow it to teach me to stop thinking first of myself. How else will I learn to see beyond the mere appearance of someone who may one day have forgotten my name? Look further, look through, says a still, small voice, and see instead the winsome beauty of a soul created by an unseen Hand. To a crucified God, it is a beauty to die for.

And for a lesser being like myself, it should be worth at least another wind.

Drowsiness begins to wrap my thoughts like a blanket. I slip gently into sleep, still wondering. Sometime in the not-so-distant future, will my own children, and their children, visit me out of affection, duty, or both? And will the grandkids, bless them, learn to play mahjongg for our amusement? One cannot know such things in advance. But we had better take good care of that table, just in case.

A Caregiver Resilience Program

Meeting Alzheimer's
Learning to Communicate and Connect

Created by
Rev. Dr. Jade C. Angelica
Founder and Director
Healing Moments for Alzheimer's
www.healingmoments.org

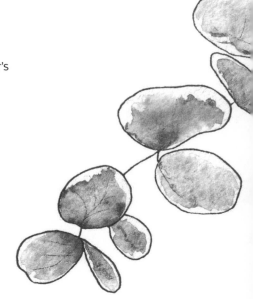

Destiny

The breeze at dawn has secrets to tell you.
Don't go back to sleep.

— Jalāl al-Dīn Rumi

I was shepherded into the Alzheimer's journey in 2001 by the diagnosis of a family member—my mother, Jeanne. At first, I did my best to avoid the whole topic, which was an especially terrifying one for me because of the potential genetic component. Both of Mom's older sisters had died from Alzheimer's disease. Avoidance was not all that difficult at the beginning because I was living in Maine and Mom lived in Iowa. As the years went on, however, it became necessary for me to actively participate in Mom's care, and that's when Destiny intervened, bringing exactly what I needed. When my Doctor of Ministry program advisor, Dr. Brita Gill-Austern, learned about my desire to care for my mother and to witness her illness from a spiritual perspective, she gave me the second edition of Dr. Stephen Post's book, *The Moral Challenge of Alzheimer Disease,* along with his article, "Alzheimer's and Grace." His words influenced me to my core. They informed, inspired, and empowered me. They guided me through difficult decision making, helped me to improve the quality of Mom's life and my own, and solidified my understanding of the inherent worth and dignity of every person—especially the deeply forgetful. He invited me into the experience of feeling a respite from the stresses of my busy life in the presence of persons living with Alzheimer's, and he taught me that kindness and love can transcend any obstacle to creating and maintaining meaningful relationships.

Through Dr. Post's example, I realized that I have a contribution to make toward the healing of the deeply forgetful and their caregivers. Ultimately, I was encouraged by him and other authors, teachers, healers, and friends to pay forward the grace I received from them by founding Healing Moments for Alzheimer's—a nonprofit organization whose mission is to benefit persons living with Alzheimer's and dementia, and their caregivers, through unique, innovative, compassionate programming that is both reflection and practical application of seeds planted in my soul by Dr. Stephen Post.

Discovery

I have also learned that it is better to be always kind than always right about time and place.

— Stephen G. Post

Although I am the founder of Healing Moments, I did not set out to develop a workshop—or to write a book (*Where Two Worlds Touch: A Spiritual Journey through Alzheimer's Disease*). The goal of my research and study was to learn and grow—intellectually, emotionally, and spiritually—in order to become a helpful companion for my mother during the time in her life when she was the most vulnerable and needed me more than ever before. The resources I created evolved through a process of ongoing discovery. Every day of my journey with Mom was about living my life in relationship with her, being attentive to the changes she was experiencing—we were experiencing—noticing her needs and joys, losses and remaining abilities, and making discovery after discovery.

Although distance facilitated my avoidance at first, two years after Mom's diagnosis she and a relative traveled to Maine to visit me. It was then that I met Alzheimer's disease, "in person," through my mother's eyes, her words, and her unedited presence. During this time together, I was deeply touched by Mom's obvious decline and what I can only describe as exquisite vulnerability. This "meeting"—which for me resembled the "I/Thou" encounters described by Martin Buber where essence meets essence (Buber 1987, 11)—opened my heart, and discoveries began flowing in.

A year later, three aspects of my life came together at the same time—like planets converging in the skies—and everything changed for Mom and for me. First, my sister, who lived with Mom, asked me to come to Iowa to take care of Mom for two weeks. Second, for the previous two years, I had been taking improvisational theatre classes. This was a terrific stretch for me because I am not the improv type. Nevertheless, I was learning to accept and advance what was offered in life; I was transforming from a frightened "no-sayer" into an adventurous "yes-sayer" (Johnstone 1992, 92); and I was, surprisingly, becoming increasingly OK not knowing what in the world was going on. The third puzzle piece that facilitated my learning and growth was the moment I made the life-altering, healing connection between improvisation and how this theatre craft can help us meet deeply forgetful persons in their worlds and make connections with them there.

My sister had asked me to come to Iowa so she could go on a camping vacation. Mom could no longer be left alone, and taking her camping the previous summer had a disastrous ending that involved the Minnesota Highway Patrol and a hospital emergency room. Because of the quality of our time together during Mom's visit to Maine and the sweet letters and conversations we had shared since then, I was eager to spend more time with her; so I enthusiastically said, "Yes" to this request. After hearing my "Yes," my sister then shared some alarming details. She said, "Mom is really uncooperative, angry, and combative. She won't eat, take her medicine, or do what I tell her to do. In order to get her to obey, you'll have to raise your voice, threaten to take her to the mental hospital, or give her the antipsychotic drugs I got from her internist." And then she added, "The drugs do make her kind of out of it for weeks, though." At this point, I became very worried, wondering, "What in the world have I said 'Yes' to?"

Sadly, I later learned that my sister's approach is common, even still. People who don't understand the disease do get frustrated and sometimes they yell, threaten, and use physical force or drugs—trying to get our dear, vulnerable, deeply forgetful loved ones living with Alzheimer's and dementia under control. For me, this approach was completely unacceptable, so I was determined to find a better way. And I did: improvisation!

During our two weeks together, Mom gave me countless opportunities to practice the improvisation techniques I had been learning in my classes. When I was able to meet Mom in her world—which is the communication technique that experts in the dementia care field, including Dr. Post, have been recommending for over thirty years—she was not the angry, combative person she was advertised to be. She was just marching to her own tune, trying to preserve her dignity, trying to communicate her needs and desires, and using her remaining, although declining, cognitive abilities. With the help of improvisation, I was able to get into step with her, and our time together went very well. We became close and compatible companions.

One improvised "meeting" with Mom that was both endearing and moving involved her sister, Milly. We had planned an outing to the nursing home to visit her friend, Martin, and when it was nearly time to go, I asked, "Mom, are you ready?"

Visibly upset by my question, she replied, "We can't go."

I responded with curiosity. "But, I thought you wanted to see Marty?"

"Not now," Mom said. "This is the time that Milly comes to visit me."

Milly died in 1991; we had planted flowers on her grave the day before. Instead of correcting Mom, and possibly demeaning her for forgetting or breaking her heart by reminding her that her beloved sister was long dead, I chose to improvise. I made the conscious choice to join Mom in her world—where we were expecting Milly. Presuming Mom's statement to be valid (according to her reality) and factoring our existing plans into the equation, I said the next logical thing. "Well, what would you think about leaving Milly a note, telling her where we are, and asking her to come inside and wait for us?"

After pausing for a moment, Mom said, "That's a good idea."

"OK." I said. "Could you get a piece of paper and a pencil, and we'll write the note?"

"Oh, yes. I'll do that." And she was off to find the paper and pencil. I wrote the note, Mom taped it to the door, and we went to visit Marty, as planned.

Improvisers would call my response "accepting and advancing the offer." Alzheimer's experts would identify this as a "therapeutic fiblette" (Raia 1999, 32), because I did not try to correct Mom with my truth or orient her into the current time and place. Spiritual teachers would call this honoring another's perspective—which helps to avoid conflict—

and accepting another's reality, Mom's reality, born out of Alzheimer's. Science informs us that this kind of radical acceptance when relating to deeply forgetful persons is one of the most effective coping techniques for relieving caregiver stress (Powers, Gallagher-Thompson, and Kraemer 2002). All these disciplines would remind us that accepting reality in the present provides the most positive springboard into the future.

Engaging in improvisation, Mom and I followed her reality into a present and a future that overflowed with love, connection, and healing. The day before I was leaving to return to Maine, Mom was able to tell me, in her own precious way, that my efforts to learn about Alzheimer's, my attempts to communicate creatively by using improvisation, and my compassionate attention had made an impression on her. She looked up at me from her chair in the living room, and said, "Will you stay and take care of me? You're kinder to me." In that moment, my heart shouted out, "Yes!"; and my yes-saying, healing adventure into Alzheimer's sprouted wings. When I returned to Maine, the birth process for the Meeting Alzheimer's workshop began to take flight.

The Workshop

The information and ideas presented in the Meeting Alzheimer's workshop are fresh, practical, applicable, and memorable. Not only did the group enjoy themselves and learn something new; most importantly, they learned techniques they can put into practice. The lessons learned by the group, and no doubt retained, will directly benefit their loved ones with memory loss. "Yes, let's" is my new motto!

— Melanie Chavin, Alzheimer's Association, Illinois Chapter

Summary of the Workshop

Uniting spirit, art, scholarship, and science, the Meeting Alzheimer's workshop is designed to improve the quality of life for deeply forgetful persons, reduce caregiver stress, and inspire a hopeful attitude for all. The intent of this programming, which is both informative and supportive, is to help individuals and communities develop a more comprehensive understanding of these diseases, and to nurture the beliefs that personal value exists and meaningful relationships remain possible throughout all the stages of Alzheimer's and other diseases with symptoms of dementia.

Using experiential methods based on improvisational theatre exercises and mindfulness practices, Meeting Alzheimer's teaches caregivers how to:

- effectively implement the recommended communication techniques of "meeting in the moment,"
- connect deeply with persons with cognitive decline via "emotional memory,"
- identify and accept the limitations and discover the gifts of Alzheimer's and dementia,
- reduce conflict, increase cooperation, and provide quality, therapeutic care.

The two-day (twelve-hour) workshop for family caregivers was the subject of a research study by the University of Iowa Department of Neurology from 2014 to 2017. The findings, published in *Alzheimer's & Dementia: Transactional and Clinical Interventions*, show that participants in this workshop experienced a significant reduction in stress, and an increase in their feelings of confidence and competence in their caregiver role over a period of at least six months (Spalding-Wilson et al. 2018). The Iowa researchers were particularly interested in studying the Meeting Alzheimer's workshop because they perceived it to be a practical application of their earlier findings about the retention of emotional memory in persons with amnesia, published in 2010 (Feinstein, Duff, and Tranel 2010), and in deeply forgetful persons with Alzheimer's published in 2014 (Guzmán-Vélez, Feinstein, and Tranel 2014). A continuing collaboration with University of Iowa researchers for further study of the workshop benefits for caregivers, as well as benefits for their deeply forgetful loved ones, is being planned, with the express intention of reaching underserved populations in rural areas.

Description of the Workshop

All of the Healing Moments for Alzheimer's experiential programs for caregivers (family, professional, and informal) translate state-of-the-art dementia care theory into practice, and are available in a variety of formats, including a didactic play, *The Forgiving & The Forgetting*. The Meeting Alzheimer's workshop formats range from a seventy-five-minute introductory/conference presentation to a twelve-hour intensive training, all of which include structured presentations, interactive experiences and educational exercises, discussion, sharing of stories and concerns, and opportunities for supportive relationship-building among participants. The shorter workshops can accommodate hundreds of participants; the twelve-hour training is limited to twenty-four. To maximize retention, content is designed to engage participants physically, intellectually, and emotionally, and is presented in ways that are energizing, enlightening, and enjoyable.

Rarely do we hear the words "Alzheimer's" and "fun" in the same sentence; therefore, some may be surprised when they hear the Meeting Alzheimer's workshop described as "fun." Although the exercises and experiences may be unexpected and seem different—possibly even a little silly at first—they coincide with specific treatment modalities such as Habilitation Therapy, Validation Therapy, Act and Commitment Therapy (ACT), Emotion Focused Therapy (EFT), and Compassion Focused Therapy (CFT), and they have been carefully selected to enhance caregiving skills. What may seem like fun on the surface is actually highly instructive programming. The improvisation exercises, in particular, are introduced incrementally, providing a non-threatening environment so as to increase participant enjoyment and success. Participants discover, as I did, that improvisation, when practiced as a craft, is not about performance or comedy, or being clever, or even inventive. Improvisation is about being authentic, welcoming the present moment, saying the next logical thing, and trusting that everything we need is already here, waiting to be discovered (LaGraffe 2012). The "first rule" of improvisation—which is to make your scene partner look good—is applicable and so essential in our relationships with the deeply forgetful.

The Habilitation Model of Alzheimer's care, developed over two decades ago by Dr. Paul Raia and Joanne Koenig Coste, identifies six domains (physical, functional, social, communication, perceptual, and behavioral) (Raia 1999, 22) where quality of life for deeply forgetful persons can be enhanced, indicating that the communication domain offers the most potential toward this goal. Accordingly, the main focus of the Meeting Alzheimer's workshop is on communicating and connecting, developing and deepening meaningful relationships, creating positive emotional interactions, and providing effective, therapeutic care that responds—as Dr. Post notes—to "needs that are chiefly relational and physical" (Post 2018).

Content of the Workshop

These are some of the major topics covered in the workshop.

Dignity and Worth

Although there are many techniques currently available to Alzheimer's caregivers, and although Healing Moments offers a unique and effective combination of techniques, now shown by research to significantly reduce caregiver stress, the Meeting Alzheimer's workshop does not begin with any technique. The words of Dr. James Ellor, gerontologist and professor of social work at Baylor University, echo the perspective of Dr. Post. Together, they have guided me to begin differently. In his essay "Celebrating the Human Spirit," Dr. Ellor wrote: "The first principle of working with a person who has Alzheimer's disease involves a value rather than a technique" (Ellor 1997, 13). In an interview, Dr. Post said, "Ultimately, my message is about the dignity and worth of deeply forgetful people, and how they merit equal consideration in the vast heterogeneity of a shared humanity" (Post 2018). In order to usher caregivers through the doorway of effective skill building, we first uncover and deconstruct the cultural conditioning that has planted ideas in many minds, having them believe that people living with Alzheimer's or other forms of dementia are gone, lost, empty shells, dead before they are dead. We replace these misconceptions by identifying and speaking for the true value of this vulnerable population, which has always been the foundation of Dr. Post's work. As he states, "Caregivers are the ones who protect and advocate for the dignity of deeply forgetful people and convey to society the message that moral inclusion in the human family does not depend on the relative strength of memory" (Post 2018). Understanding and respecting their value and standing in solidarity with their dignity are the first and necessary ingredients of quality care. Throughout the workshop, concrete suggestions, encouragement, and support for protective actions and advocacy are provided in practical ways.

Observing

Using mindfulness meditation techniques, caregivers practice turning their attention to the present moment, and then acknowledge and share what they have noticed. Most experience this eight minutes of silent observation to be quite relaxing, and although this is a wonderful outcome, it's not the primary point of the experience. Given the declining abilities that are characteristic of Alzheimer's disease and other diseases of dementia, our skills of observation will be crucial to the well-being of the deeply forgetful, since they will not always be the best reporters of what is happening for and to them. It is equally necessary that caregivers observe ourselves, since the demands on our time, energy, patience, problem-solving abilities, and creativity are enormous. Because the focus of the workshop is highly relational, the needs, challenges, and contributions of those in relationships with the deeply forgetful are held in the light, stressing self-care as a significant component of successful caregiving. This point circles us back to the relaxation of body and spirit that can result from pausing in a quiet environment, breathing, and attempting to calm our minds for as few as five minutes. Even a brief mindful pause, done regularly, can lead to health benefits and be an effective method for enhancing emotional awareness, compassion, and empathy. However, since most of us (caregivers, especially) are more often active than we are sitting and breathing in a quiet place, the workshop takes our mindfulness practice into active exercises that strengthen caregivers' skills of observation on physical (outward) and emotional (inward) levels.

The Importance of Acceptance

Family members of deeply forgetful persons often feel hurt and frustrated when their loved ones don't remember their names—or if and how they are related. Caregivers can get tormented by a painful cycle, giving them hope for recovery one day when their deeply forgetful loved ones seem oriented in the present, and then catapulted into despair the next day when their loved ones are clearly living in the past. It happens often that both family and professional caregivers become angry, blaming their loved ones (or care center residents) for behaviors such as repeating or forgetting or emotional outbursts, manifested by the predictable progression of Alzheimer's or other degenerative brain diseases. These reactions by caregivers highlight the urgent priority of implementing the coping technique of accepting what is. The Meeting Alzheimer's workshop focuses on acceptance throughout, introducing, exploring, and practicing this simple definition by Nathaniel Brandon: "Experiencing without denial or avoidance, that a fact is a fact." Acceptance in relationship to the deeply forgetful is about respecting others' realities, that their facts are their facts—and valid. In order for caregivers to reach true acceptance, the path often takes them through a thorny patch of resistance. Therefore, we also explore the many reasons for resistance, most of which are rooted in fear. For example, fear of the unknown; fear of letting go of control; fear of fully embracing the losses; fear of encouraging "wrong" realities; fear of criticism for taking an alternative and creative approach; fear of seeming or feeling like a failure for not being able to do it all. To overcome resistance, we offer exercises that invite participants to practice flexibility, meet the unknown with courage, adjust expectations, and fully engage with the realities of the diseases of dementia. As caregivers engage in the process of meeting their fears and pain, we introduce the guiding light of Indian poet Rabindranath Tagore: "Let me not pray to be sheltered from dangers, but to be fearless in facing them. Let me not beg for the stilling of my pain, but for the heart to conquer it."

Communicating and Connecting

The most important domain for improving quality of life for deeply forgetful persons, effective communication training, is consistently woven throughout the workshop. Scripted scenes from real life, topic-specific presentations, and exercises drawn from mindfulness meditation and improvisation deliver information about and provide practice for:

- being present in *their* moments;
- letting go of the need for control;
- accepting the realities and limitations that accompany cognitive decline;
- learning how healing can happen in the absence of cure; pushing back at the cultural hopelessness that wages "war" against dementia, which is perceived as "the worst condition imaginable" (Post 2018);
- developing a hopeful attitude by identifying ways both caregivers and the deeply forgetful can—and do—make a difference in each other's lives;
- maintaining self-esteem for people who are losing so much;
- and—most importantly—recognizing and celebrating all that remains.

During the times in the workshop set aside for sharing stories, we deliberately raise up and celebrate those small and precious moments where connection happens, and we experience joy. These are the moments that energize us for the long term, and that we will remember forever.

Managing Difficult Behaviors

Throughout the workshop, information coalesces and exercises build on one another in ways that are designed to teach caregivers how to interact with deeply forgetful persons in order to increase cooperation, as well as providing caregivers with opportunities to truly feel empathy and compassion for others. Specific experiences and scripted scenes of actual encounters provide practice in saying "Yes, let's" instead of "No, you can't," and noticing and feeling the consequences that result from both responses. Caregivers need teaching in this important practice of yes-saying because for many of us it does not come naturally; others resist, believing that saying "Yes" to an altered reality is lying, which they consider both undignified and immoral based on religious principles. The therapeutic nature of saying "Yes," and the recommendation of experts to do this is emphasized. Also emphasized is the importance of accepting that deeply forgetful persons are trying to communicate with us—even when they can no longer speak. Researchers consider them to be semiotic subjects who communicate using signs and symbols (Millett 2011, 12). What looks like an acting-out behavior is often actually an effort to communicate! It is up to attentive, observant caregivers to seek to understand.

Verbal and Nonverbal Communication

Citing the research of Dr. Edmarie Guzmán-Vélez and the University of Iowa Department of Neurology, participants learn about the retention of emotional memory by deeply forgetful persons. This groundbreaking research confirms through science what observant caregivers have known all along:

- "Heart Memories" last for long periods of time even when the event that caused the feeling cannot be recalled (Guzmán-Vélez, Feinstein, and Tranel 2014; Eder 1984).
- Emotions are what deeply forgetful persons with Alzheimer's are "good at" (Raia 1999, 31).
- Emotions remain throughout all the stages of the disease.

Building on skills practiced earlier in the workshop, caregivers learn to see and hear beneath failing words in order to recognize and connect with the emotions being expressed. Since deeply forgetful persons cannot recall what caused a feeling, process their emotions, or soothe themselves when they are upset, another important goal for quality Alzheimer's caregiving is to create opportunities for more positive emotions to be experienced, and especially to avoid creating painful feelings. However, when painful feelings do emerge, it is necessary for caregivers to know how to offer consolation and how to relieve distress in order to effectively meet the deeply forgetful in their emotional experiences. Workshop participants discuss, learn about, and practice techniques for communicating and connecting that can successfully further these goals.

Caregiver Recognition and Appreciation

Caregivers do not always or often receive appreciation from deeply forgetful persons—not because they are not appreciated, but because persons with all forms of progressive dementia will eventually lose the ability to initiate this kind of relational communication. One of the most heart-opening exercises in the Meeting Alzheimer's workshop gives participants an opportunity to appreciate each other. Strangers, most of them, bond sincerely through a shared understanding of the challenges and heartbreaks they encounter and endure as caregivers. Each participant is invited to take the hands of another caregiver, make eye contact, and share those longed-for words, "I appreciate you." They can say this to each other with integrity because they know how hard every caregiver is working and trying. Their partners in this exercise graciously receive this gift of appreciation, replying with the words, "I know." Done quietly and reverently, the power of this exchange can touch tender places in the soul.

Throughout my journey through Alzheimer's, friends and authors helped me to understand why this exercise was so important to include in the workshop. A close friend of mine, Sister Mary Owen, lived in Wisconsin, and was in her eighties when I had the joy of meeting her. For most of her career she worked as a nurse, and she knew the statistics about Alzheimer's affecting one-third of the people in the United States over eighty-five. She felt afraid that she might get it. She was not alone in this fear. Research indicates that Americans are more afraid of getting Alzheimer's disease than they are of dying. Sister Mary Owen shared her fears with one of her sisters, whose calming reply reflects the motivation for all those involved in the Healing Moments work. She said, "If you had someone who understood the disease to take really good care of you, maybe it wouldn't be so bad." As I pondered this comment, I stumbled upon a quote by author Martha Beck that enlightens us about an aspect of human nature as it relates to Alzheimer's care. "When frightened, all primates—except humans—will seek out a safe place. Humans will seek out a safe person" (Beck 2005). Dr. Post's wisdom and words helped me to see that family caregivers are truly the unsung heroes—the safe persons—in the midst of the Alzheimer's epidemic. "Written words cannot approximate the power of the caregiver's story in inspiring us all to touch other human beings, no matter how much cognitive power they have lost, and thereby stretch the limits of our humanity in love" (Post 2000, 142). By including caregiver appreciation within the context of the Meeting Alzheimer's workshop, our hope is that participants will embody the actuality of how much their efforts to learn to be competent, confident, and compassionate caregivers are appreciated, even though their loved ones cannot always say it.

Transformation

The person with Alzheimer's is eventually swept away, while caregivers look back and feel forever changed by their experience.

— Stephen G. Post

Since my mother died in January 2011, some of my best days have been with caregivers at the Meeting Alzheimer's workshops. The solid foundation of the workshop is unquestionably to help caregivers help themselves and their loved ones on the journey through Alzheimer's disease. But those who choose to dig through this foundation of information, practicalities, and techniques will discover the invitation Dr. Post extended to me—to be changed by this journey. Seen from the surface, or even the modern medical model, the mindfulness experiences in the workshop could be interpreted solely as ways for caregivers to improve their own wellness or coping during a difficult time. But as a transformational practice, mindfulness is completely relational and ethical. "Its fruits are not wellness, personal longevity or neuroplasticity. They are compassion, equanimity, and love" (Bourgeault 2016, 112). Similarly, the present-moment function of improvisation mirrors these fruits. In addition, the most challenging invitation from the craft of improvisation, letting go of the need to be right, the need to control, and even the need to know what's next, in order to be right here, right now in relatedness with our deeply forgetful loved ones, can help us to shift from being no-sayers to yes-sayers. Through this shift, it is possible to transform the way we engage with everyone and the world, ultimately reducing the pain we experience in all areas of our lives from resisting what is.

What a joy it has been, and is, for me to lead people along this path of transformation—pointing out the way as we travel together. It is so deeply rewarding to welcome weeping caregivers to the workshop; to send them home after a day, or two days, radiating hope and empowerment; and then to hear weeks, months, and years later about the impact of the workshop. One week after attending the workshop, Leonora, primary caregiver for her father, Leo, wrote: "I'm still feeling great—very optimistic and upbeat regarding the challenges I am facing with my father." One month later she wrote: "I'm enjoying my father's company more and more. I'm noticing he does much better when I show concern about his feelings. It actually seems he remembers more." Two years later she wrote: "My father is declining. He can no longer walk, and when he talks nothing makes sense, but we just give him the respect and care he deserves, and make sure he's happy" (Leonora 2007-2009).

At the beginning of the workshop caregivers practice mindfulness while listening to a song, paying attention to their feelings. A man in his eighties, who was caregiver for his wife, began to cry. He was embarrassed. I sat by him, reassuring him that all of him was welcome, including his tears. He told me he thought he should leave. I supported his choice, reassured him that the rest of the day would not be as emotional, and suggested that perhaps he would like to stay for a while and see. He stayed for the entire time. At the end of the workshop, he took me aside. With a smile and a twinkle, he said, "I really think I can do this now."

Although I have been leading these workshops for over twelve years, I am always surprised and delighted to witness the fervor with which mature, reserved, sometimes hesitant fifty-, sixty-, seventy-, and eighty-year-old men and women open themselves to the relationship-building possibilities available through improvisation and mindfulness. Together we laugh, learn, and open our minds and hearts; together we change. At the end of the workshop, participants are given the opportunity to share an important something they learned and will take home with them. Ben, one of those men in his late seventies, caregiver for his wife, said simply. "I am different now. I am a different person. Thank you so much."

For me, personally, the transformation happened without me actually realizing it was underway. I first recognized and named it about six months after Mom died, in response to a passing comment made by a colleague. We had been working together on the Healing Moments CD, *Meeting Alzheimer's: Companionship on the Journey*, and I took a proof copy of the music to her home so we could listen together. As I was leaving, she stopped me and said, "You are such an unusual combination of qualities—you are both really organized and really sweet." Hearing this, I paused to receive and consider her observations; and then said what I knew to be true. "I used to just be organized. Caring for Mom made me sweet." Dr. Post's prediction had come true for me. By implementing the techniques I now have the honor of sharing with other caregivers, I was forever changed.

Rev. Dr. Jade C. Angelica

Jade Angelica is a sojourner from the land of Alzheimer's bearing witness that all there is not lost. Her testimony is even more outrageous: we can experience in that far country depths of being alive, and in love, that the worlds of perfect health may never understand.

— Michael Verde, Founder and Director, Memory Bridge

Rev. Dr. Jade Angelica designs workshops, services, and trainings for Healing Moments for Alzheimer's (www.healingmoments.org) and offers presentations throughout the country. In addition, Jade offers spiritual direction for individuals and groups. She is the author of *Where Two Worlds Touch: A Spiritual Journey Through Alzheimer's Disease* and *Meeting Alzheimer's: Companionship on the Journey*, currently available in audio format. She is also the author of the play *The Forgiving & The Forgetting: Hope and Healing for Alzheimer's*. Her articles have appeared in *The Journal of Reli-*

gion, *Spirituality and Aging, The Journal of Pastoral Care & Counseling, Presence, The World, The National Catholic Reporter,* and *The Huffington Post.* Her essay "Through My Eyes" is included in *Seasons of Caring: Meditations for Alzheimer's and Dementia Caregivers,* an interfaith book published by Clergy-AgainstAlzheimer's Network.

Jade's education and training include a master of divinity from Harvard Divinity School, a certificate from the Shalem Institute Spiritual Guidance Program, a doctor of ministry in faith, health and spirituality from Andover Newton Theological School, and a diploma from Improv Boston University that deems her "perfectly OK not knowing what in the world is going on!"

Jade's most important and most rewarding ministry to date has been caring for her mother, Jeanne, who died from Alzheimer's in 2011.

She may be reached at jadeangelica@gmail.com.

REFERENCES

Beck, M. 2005. *Finding Your Own North Star: Claiming the Life You Were Meant to Live,* unabridged edition. Boulder, CO: Sounds True Publishing, compact disc.

Bourgeault, C. 2016. *The Heart of Centering Prayer: Nondual Christianity in Theory and Practice.* Boulder, CO: Shambhala.

Buber, M. 1987 (originally published 1958). *I and Thou,* 2nd ed. R. G. Smith, trans. New York: Scribner Classic/Collier Books.

Eder, Louise. 1984. "Heart Memories." The poem was first published in the newsletter of the Kansas City Association for Alzheimer's and Related Dementias.

Ellor, J. W. 1997. "Celebrating the Human Spirit." In *God Never Forgets: Faith, Hope and Alzheimer's Disease,* edited by D. K. McKim, 1-20. Louisville, KY: Westminster John Knox Press.

Feinstein, J., M. Duff, and D. Tranel. 2010. "Sustained Experience of Emotion after Loss of Memory in Patients with Amnesia." *PNAS/Proceedings of the National Academy of Science of the United States of America* 107 (17): 7674-7679.

Guzmán-Vélez, E., J. Feinstein, and D. Tranel. 2014. "Feelings without Memory in Alzheimer Disease." *Cognitive Behavioral Neurology* 27 (3): 117-127.

Johnstone, K. 1992. *IMPRO: Improvisation and The Theatre.* New York: Routledge.

LaGraffe, D. 2012. Lights Up Improvisation, Portland, ME. Interview with author J. Angelica.

Leonora. 2007-2009. Emails to author J. Angelica from workshop participant Leonora.

Millett, S. 2011. "Self and Embodiment: A Biophenomenological Approach to Dementia." *Dementia* 10, no. 4 (November 2011): 509-522. https://doi.org/10.1177/1471301211409374.

Post, S. G. 2000. *The Moral Challenge of Alzheimer Disease: Ethical Issues from Diagnosis to Dying,* 2nd ed. Baltimore: Johns Hopkins University Press.

———. 2018. Interview with author J. Angelica.

Powers, D. V., D. Gallagher-Thompson, and H. C. Kraemer. 2002. "Coping and Depression in Alzheimer's Caregivers: Longitudinal Evidence of Stability." *Journal of Gerontology: Psychological Sciences* 57B (3): 205-211. A 2015 study includes a survey of research on various coping styles: https://www.ncbi.nlm.nih.gov/pmc/articles/PMC4845636/.

Raia, P. 1999. "Habilitation Therapy: A New Starscape." In *Enhancing the Quality of Life in Advanced Dementia,* edited by L. Volcer and L. Bloom-Charette, 21-37. Philadelphia: Brunner/Mazel.

Spalding-Wilson, K., E. Guzmán-Vélez, J. Angelica, K. Wiggs, A. Savransky, and D. Tranel. 2018. "A Novel Two-Day Intervention Reduces Stress in Caregivers of Persons with Dementia." *Alzheimer's & Dementia: Transactional Research and Clinical Interventions* 4:450-460. https://www.ncbi.nlm.nih.gov/pmc/articles/PMC6153380.

references

Adkins, R. 1998. "Husband of Kevorkian Patient Speaks Out." *Advances: National Newsletter of the Alzheimer's Disease and Related Disorders Association, Inc.* (Chicago) 18 (1): 2.

Ahronheim, J. C., M. Mulvihill, and C. Sieger. 2001. "State Practice Variations in the Use of Tube Feeding for Nursing Home Residents with Severe Cognitive Impairment." *Journal of the American Geriatrics Society* 49: 148-152.

Alexander, L. 1949. "Medicine under the Nazis." *New England Journal of Medicine* 241 (2): 39-47.

Algase, D. L. 1992. "A Century of Progress: Today's Strategies for Responding to Wandering Behavior." *Journal of Gerontological Nursing* 18 (11): 28-34.

Alzheimer's Disease Association. 2001. *Ethical Issues in Alzheimer's Disease*. Chicago: Alzheimer's Disease Association.

American Geriatrics Society. 2014. "American Geriatrics Society Feeding Tubes in Advanced Dementia Position Statement." *Journal of the American Geriatrics Society* 62:1590-1593.

Ariyoshi, S. 1984. *The Twilight Years*. New York: Kodansha International.

Augustine, St. 1961. *Confessions*. Translated by R. S. Pine-Coffin. Harmondsworth, UK: Penguin Classics.

Barstow, C., B. Shahan, and M. Roberts. 2018. "Evaluating Medical Decision-Making Capacity in Practice." *American Family Physician* 98 (1): 40-46.

Batthyany, A., and B. Greyson. 2020. "Spontaneous Remission of Dementia before Death: Results from a Study on Paradoxical Lucidity." *Psychology of Consciousness: Theory, Research, and Practice*, a Journal of the American Psychological Association. https://doi.org/10.1037/cns0000259.

Beach, M. C., T. Inui, and Relationship-Centered Care Research Network. 2006. "Relationship-Centered Care. A Constructive Reframing." *Journal of General Internal Medicine* 21 suppl. 1: S3–S8. doi: 10.1111/j.1525-1497.2006.00302.x.

Beauchamp, T. L., and J. F. Childress. 2013. *Principles of Biomedical Ethics.* New York: Oxford University Press.

Bell, C., E. Somogyi-Zalud, and K. Masaki. 2008. "Factors Associated with Physician Decision-Making in Starting Tube Feeding." *Journal of Palliative Medicine* 11 (6): 915–922.

Bergson, H. 1994 (originally published 1896). *Matter and Memory: An Essay on the Relation of Body and Spirit.* New York: Zone Books.

Berkovich, S. Y. 1993. "On the Information Processing Capabilities of the Brain: Shifting the Paradigm." *Nanobiology* 2:99–107.

Berrios, G. E., and M. Mohanna. 1990. "Durkheim and French Psychiatric Views on Suicide during the Nineteenth Century: A Conceptual History." *British Journal of Psychiatry* 156:1–9.

Binstock, R. H., S. G. Post, and P. J. Whitehouse, eds. 1992. *Dementia and Aging: Ethics, Values and Policy Choices.* Baltimore: Johns Hopkins University Press.

Brady, T. F., T. Konkle, G. A. Alvarez, and A. Oliva. 2008. "Visual Long-Term Memory Has a Massive Storage Capacity for Object Details." *Proceedings of the National Academy of Sciences* 105:14325–14329.

Braun, U. K., L. Rabeneck, and L. B. McCullough. 2005. "Decreasing Use of Percutaneous Endoscopic Gastrostomy Tube Feeding for Veterans with Dementia—Racial Differences Remain." *Journal of the American Geriatrics Society* 53:242–248.

Brown, W., N. Murphy, and H. N. Malony, eds. 1998. *Whatever Happened to the Soul? Scientific and Theological Portraits of Human Nature.* Philadelphia: Fortress Press.

Brudney, D. 2009. "Choosing for Another: Beyond Autonomy and Best Interests." *Hastings Center Report* 39 (2): 31–37.

Buchanan, A. E., and D. W. Brock. 1990. *Deciding for Others: The Ethics of Surrogate Decision Making.* New York: Cambridge University Press.

Cervo, F. A., L. Bryan, and S. Farber. 2006. "To PEG or Not to PEG: A Review of Evidence for Placing Feeding Tubes in Advanced Dementia and the Decision-Making Process." *Geriatrics* 61 (6): 30–35.

Cheng, S. T., E. Mak, H. Fung, T. Kwok, D. Lee, and L. Lam. 2017. "Benefit-Finding and Effect on Caregiver Depression: A Double-Blind Randomized Controlled Trial." *Journal of Consulting and Clinical Psychology* 85 (5): 521–529.

Cheng, S. T., E. Mak, R. Lau, N. Ng, and L. Lam. 2016. "Voices of Alzheimer Caregivers on Positive Aspects of Caregiving." *The Gerontologist* 56 (3): 451-460.

Chicoine, B., D. McGuire, and S. Rubin. 1998. "Adults with Down Syndrome: Specialty Clinic Perspectives." In *Dementia, Aging, and Intellectual Disabilities: A Handbook*, edited by M. P. Janicki and A. J. Dalton, 89-97. New York: Brunner/Mazel.

Clarke, C., and E. Wolverson. 2016. "Hope and Dementia." In *Positive Psychology Approaches to Dementia*, edited by C. Clarke and E. Wolverson, 88-109. Philadelphia: Jessica Kingsley Publishers.

Cohen, C. A., P. J. Whitehouse, S. G. Post, S. A. Gauthier, and L. LeDuc. 1999. "Ethical Issues in Alzheimer Disease: The Experience of a National Alzheimer Society Task Force." *Alzheimer Disease and Associated Disorders* 13 (2): 66-70.

Cohen-Mansfield, J., P. Werner, M. S. Marx, and L. Freedman. 1991. "Two Studies of Pacing in the Nursing Home." *Journals of Gerontology* 46 (3): M77-M83.

Courtney, C. 2004. "Long-Term Donepezil Treatment in 565 Patients with Alzheimer's Disease (AD2000): Randomised Double-Blind Trial." *Lancet* 363 (9427): 2105-2115.

Cutler, N. R., L. L. Heston, P. Davies, J. V. Haxby, and M. P. Shapiro. 1985. "Alzheimer's Disease and Down's Syndrome: New Insights." *Annals of Internal Medicine* 103:566-578.

Daly, R. L., F. Bunn, and C. Goodman. 2018. "Shared Decision-Making for People Living with Dementia in Extended Care Settings: A Systematic Review." *British Medical Journal Open* 8:e018977. doi:10.1135/bmjopen-2017001897.

de Beaufort, I., and S. V. de Vathorst. 2016. "Dementia and Assisted Suicide and Euthanasia." *Journal of Neurology* 263:1463-1467.

de Oliveira, M. F., F. C. G. Pinto, K. Nishikuni, R. V. Botelho, A. M. Lima, and J. M. Rotta. 2012. "Revisiting Hydrocephalus as a Model to Study Brain Resilience." *Frontiers in Human Neuroscience* 5:181.

Detering, K. M., A. D. Hancock, M. C. Reade, and W. Silvester. 2010. "The Impact of Advance Care Planning on End of Life Care in Elderly Patients: A Randomized Controlled Trial." *British Medical Journal* 340: c1315.

Devi, G. 2017. *The Spectrum of Hope: An Optimistic and New Approach to Alzheimer's Disease and Other Dementias.* New York: Workman.

de Wachter, M. A. M. 1992. "Euthanasia in the Netherlands." *Hastings Center Report* 22 (2): 23-30.

DiGiovanni, L. 1978. "The Elderly Retarded: A Little-Known Group." *The Gerontologist* 18:262–268.

Doi, T. 1971. *The Anatomy of Dependence.* Tokyo: Kodansha International.

Drachman, D. A. 1988. "Who May Drive? Who May Not? Who Shall Decide?" *Annals of Neurology* 24:178–187.

Dresser, R. 2017. "On Legalizing Physician-Assisted Death for Dementia." *The Hastings Center Report* (July–August): 5–6.

Durkheim, E. 2005 (originally published 1897). *Suicide: A Study in Sociology*, translated by J. A. Spaulding and G. Simpson. London: Routledge.

Evenhuis, H. M. 1990. "The Natural History of Dementia in Down's Syndrome." *Archives of Neurology* 47:263–267.

Farina, N., T. Page, S. Daley, A. Brown, A. Bowling, and T. Basset. 2017. "Factors Associated with the Quality of Life of Family Carers of People with Dementia: A Systematic Review." *Alzheimer's & Dementia* 13:572–581.

Fazio, S. 2008. *The Enduring Self in People with Alzheimer's: Getting to the Heart of Individualized Care.* Baltimore: Health Professions Press.

Feuillet, L., H. Dufour, and J. Pelletier. 2007. "Brain of a White-Collar Worker." *Lancet* 370:262.

Finucane, T. E., C. Christmas, and K. Travis. 1999. "Tube Feeding in Patients with Advanced Dementia: A Review of the Evidence." *Journal of the American Medical Association* 282:1365–1370.

Foley, J. M., and S. G. Post. 1993. "Ethical Issues in Dementia." In *Handbook of Dementing Illnesses*, edited by John C. Morris, 53–59. New York: Marcel Dekker.

Forsdyke, D. R. 2015. "Wittgenstein's Certainty Is Uncertain: Brain Scans of Cured Hydrocephalics Challenge Cherished Assumptions." *Biological Theory* 10:336–342.

Fusi, S., and D. R. Abbott. 2007. "Limits on Memory Storage Capacity of Bounded Synapsis." *Nature Neuroscience* 10:485–492.

Gauderer, M. 1999. "Twenty Years of Percutaneous Endoscopic Gastrostomy: Origin and Evolution of a Concept and Its Expanded Applications." *Gastrointestinal Endoscopy* 50 (6): 879–883.

Gauderer, M., and J. L. Ponsky. 1981. "A Simplified Technique for Constructing a Tube Feeding Gastrostomy." *Surgery in Gynecology and Obstetrics* 152:83–85.

Gawande, A. 2014. *Being Mortal: Medicine and What Happens in the End.* New York: Metropolitan Books.

Gillick, M. R. 2000. "Rethinking the Role of Tube Feeding in Patients with

Advanced Dementia." *New England Journal of Medicine* 342 (3): 206-210.

Gjerdingen, D. K., J. A. Neff, M. Wang, and K. Chaloner. 1999. "Older Persons' Opinions about Life-Sustaining Procedures in the Face of Dementia." *Archives of Family Medicine* 8:421-425.

Goodman, E. 2014. "It's Always Too Soon Until It's Too Late: Advance Care Planning with Alzheimer's." *Health Affairs Blog.* April 10, 2014. doi:10.1377/hblog20140410.038393.

Groopman, J. 2005. *The Anatomy of Hope: How People Prevail in the Face of Illness.* New York: Random House.

Gwyther, L. P., and D. G. Blazer. 1984. "Family Therapy and the Dementia Patient." *American Family Physician* 29 (5): 149-156.

Hadjistavropoulos, T., T. D. Fitzgerald, and G. P. Marchildon. 2010. "Practice Guidelines for Assessing Pain in Older Persons with Dementia Residing in Long-Term Care Facilities." *Physiotherapy Canada* 62 (2): 104-113.

Hadjistavropoulos, T., K. Herr, K. M. Prkachin, K. D. Craig, S. J. Gibson, A. Lukas, and J. H. Smith. 2014. "Pain Assessment in Elderly Adults with Dementia." *The Lancet Neurology* 13 (12): 1216-1227.

Hanson, L. C., J. M. Garrett, and C. Lewis. 2008. "Physicians' Expectations of Benefit from Tube Feeding." *Journal of Palliative Medicine* 11 (8): 1130-1134.

Hart, S. 1997. *Lady from the Center: A Guide to the Alzheimer's Universe.* York, Canada: Alzheimer Society of York.

Hedge, S., and R. Ellajosuyla. 2016. "Capacity Issues and Decision-Making in Dementia." *Annals of Indian Academy of Neurology* 19, suppl. 1: S34-S39.

Helme, T. 1993. "'A Special Defence': A Psychiatric Approach to Formalising Euthanasia." *British Journal of Psychiatry* 163:456-466.

High, D. M., P. J. Whitehouse, and S. G. Post [with Directors of the NIA Alzheimer's Disease Research Centers and Alzheimer's Disease Centers]. 1994. "Guidelines for Addressing Ethical and Legal Issues in Alzheimer Disease Research." *Alzheimer Disease & Associated Disorders* 8, suppl. 4: 66-74.

Hoblitzelle, O. 2008. *Ten Thousand Joys & Ten Thousand Sorrows: A Couple's Journey through Alzheimer's.* New York: Penguin.

Howard, H., R. McShane, D. M. James-Lindesay, and C. Ritchie. 2012. "Donepezil and Memantine for Moderate-to-Severe Alzheimer's Disease." *New England Journal of Medicine* 366:893-903.

Hughes, J. C. 2006. "Beyond Hypercognitivism: A Philosophical Basis for Good Quality Palliative Care in Dementia." *Les Cahiers de la Fondation Mederic Alzheimer* 2:17-23.

———. 2014. *How We Think about Dementia: Personhood, Rights, the Arts and What They Mean for Care*. London: Jessica Kingsley Publishers.

Humphry, D. 1991. *Final Exit: The Practicalities of Self-Deliverance and Assisted Suicide for the Dying*. Eugene, OR: Hemlock Society.

Ikels, C. 1998. "The Experience of Dementia in China." *Culture, Medicine and Psychiatry* 22:257-283.

Ises, E., H. van Gennip, W. Roeline, M. G. Oosertveld-Vlug, D. L. Williams, B. D. Onwuteaka-Philipsen. 2016. "How Dementia Affects Dignity: A Qualitative Study on the Perspective of Individuals with Mild and Moderate Dementia." *Journals of Gerontology: Social Sciences* 71 (3): 491-501.

Janata, P. 2009. "The Neural Architecture of Music-Evoked Autobiographical Memories." *Cerebral Cortex* 9:2579-2594.

Janicki, M. P. 1991. *Building the Future: Planning and Community Development in Aging and Developmental Disabilities*. Albany, NY: Office of Mental Retardation and Development.

Jensen, C. J., and J. Inker. 2014. "Strengthening the Dementia Care Trial: Identifying Knowledge Gaps and Linking to Resources." *American Journal of Alzheimer's Disease & Other Dementias* 30 (3): 268-275.

Jervis, G. A. 1948. "Early Senile Dementia in Mongoloid Idiocy." *American Journal of Psychiatry* 105:102-106.

Karlawish, J. H. T. 2003. "Research Involving Cognitively Impaired Adults." *New England Journal of Medicine* 348 (14): 1389-1392.

Kastenbaum, R. 1992. "Death, Suicide, and the Older Adult." In *Suicide and the Older Adult*, edited by A. A. Leenaars, R. W. Maris, J. L. McIntosh, and J. Richman, 1-14. New York: Guilford Press.

Kelly, E. F., A. Crabtree, and P. Marshall, eds. 2015. *Beyond Physicalism: Toward the Reconciliation of Science and Spirituality*. Lanham, MD: Rowman & Littlefield.

Kittay, E. F. 2019. *Learning from My Daughter: The Value and Care of Disabled Minds*. New York: Oxford University Press.

Kittay, E., and L. Carlson. 2010. *Cognitive Disability and Its Challenges to Moral Philosophy*. Oxford: Wiley-Blackwell.

Kitwood, T. 1997. *Dementia Reconsidered: The Person Comes First*. Buckingham, UK: Open University Press.

Knapp, M. J., D. S. Knopman, and P. R. Solomon. 1994. "A 30-Week Randomized Controlled Trial of High-Dose Tacrine in Patients with Alzheimer's Disease." *Journal of the American Medical Association* 271 (13): 985-991.

Komiya, K., H. Ishii, and S. Teramoto. 2012. "Medical Professionals' Attitudes toward Tube Feeding for Themselves or Their Families: A Multicenter Survey in Japan." *Journal of Palliative Medicine* 15 (5): 561-566.

Kooten, J. V., M. Smalbrugge, J. C. Wouden, M. L. Stek, and C. M. Hertogh. 2017. "Prevalence of Pain in Nursing Home Residents: The Role of Dementia Stage and Dementia Subtypes." *Journal of the American Medical Directors Association* 18 (6): 522-527.

Koppelman, E. R. 2002. "Dementia and Dignity: Towards a New Method of Surrogate Decision Making." *Journal of Medicine and Philosophy* 27 (1): 65-85.

Lavin, C., and K. J. Goka. 1999. *Older Adults with Developmental Disabilities.* Amityville, NY: Baywood Publishing.

Lennox, A., H. Karlinsky, W. Meschino, J. A. Buchanan, M. E. Percy, and J. M. Berg. 1994. "Molecular Genetic Predictive Testing for Alzheimer's Disease: Deliberations and Preliminary Recommendations." *Alzheimer Disease and Associated Disorders* 8 (2): 126-147.

Leo, R. J. 1999. "Competency and the Capacity to Make Treatment Decisions: A Primer for Primary Care Physicians." *Primary Care Companion to the Journal of Clinical Psychiatry* 1 (5): 131-141. doi: 10.4088/pcc.v01n0501.

Lo, B. 1990. "Assessing Decision-Making Capacity." *Law, Medicine and Health Care: Law and Aging* 18 (3): 193-201.

Long, N. G. K., E. S. Kim, Y. Chen, M. F. Wilson, E. L. Worthington, and T. J. VanderWeele. 2020. "The Role of Hope in Subsequent Health and Well-Being for Old Adults: An Outcome-Wide Longitudinal Approach." *Global Epidemiology* 2. https://doi.org/10.1016/j.gloepi.2020.100018.

Luckasson, R., D. Coulter, E. Polloway, S. Reiss, R. Schalock, M. Snell, D. Spitalnik, and J. Stark. 1995. *Mental Retardation: Definitions, Classifications, and Systems of Support.* Washington, DC: American Association of Mental Retardation.

Mace, N. L., and P. V. Rabins. 2021. *The 36-Hour Day*, 7th ed. Baltimore: Johns Hopkins University Press.

MacIntyre, A. 1999. *Dependent Rational Animals: Why Human Beings Need the Virtues.* Chicago: Open Court.

Martin, R. J., and P. J. Whitehouse. 1990. "The Clinical Care of Patients with Dementia." In *Dementia Care: Patient, Family, and Community*, edited by N. L. Mace, 22-31. Baltimore: Johns Hopkins University Press.

Mashour, G. A., L. Frank, A. Batthyany, A. M. Kolanowski, M. Nahm, D. Schulman-Green, B. Greyson, S. Pakhomov, J. Karlawish, and R. C. Shah. 2019.

"Paradoxical Lucidity: A Potential Paradigm Shift for the Neurobiology and Treatment of Severe Dementias." *Alzheimer's & Dementia* 15:1107-1114.

McNamara, E., and N. Kennedy. 2001. "Tube Feeding Patients with Advanced Dementia: An Ethical Dilemma." *Proceedings of the Nutrition Society* 60: 179-185.

Meier, D. E., J. C. Ahronheim, and J. Morris. 2001. "High Short-Term Mortality in Hospitalized Patients with Advanced Dementia: A Lack of Benefit of Tube Feeding." *Archives of Internal Medicine* 161 (4): 594-599.

Mendiratta, P., J. M. Tilford, and P. Prodhan. 2003. "Trends in Percutaneous Endoscopic Gastrostomy Placement in the Elderly from 1993 to 2003." *American Journal of Alzheimer's Disease & Other Dementias* 27 (8): 609-613.

Mitchell, S. 2004. "Dying with Advanced Dementia in the Nursing Home." *Archives of Internal Medicine* 164:321-326.

Mitchell, S. L., J. M. Teno, and D. K. Kiely. 2009. "The Clinical Course of Advanced Dementia." *New England Journal of Medicine* 361 (16): 1529-1538.

Muller-Hill, B. 1988. *Murderous Science: Elimination by Scientific Selection of Jews, Gypsies, and Others: Germany 1933-1945.* New York: Oxford University Press.

Nagel, T. 2012. *Mind and Cosmos: Why the Materialist Neo-Darwinian Conception of Nature Is Almost Certainly False.* New York: Oxford University Press.

Nahm, M. 2009. "Terminal Lucidity in People with Mental Illness and Other Mental Disability: An Overview and Implications for Possible Explanatory Models." *Journal of Near-Death Studies* 28 (2): 87.

Nahm, M., and B. Greyson. 2009. "Terminal Lucidity in Patients with Chronic Schizophrenia and Dementia." *The Journal of Nervous and Mental Disease* 197 (12): 942-944.

Nahm, M., B. Greyson, W. E. Kelly, and E. Haraldsson. 2012. "Terminal Lucidity: A Review and a Case Collection." *Archives of Gerontology and Geriatrics* 55 (1): 138-142.

Nakanishi, M., and K. Hattor. 2014. "Percutaneous Endoscopic Gastrostomy (PEG) Tubes Are Placed in Elderly Adults in Japan with Advanced Dementia Regardless of Expectation of Improvement in Quality of Life." *The Journal of Nutrition, Health & Aging* 18 (5): 503-510.

National Institutes of Health. 2010. *Final Panel Statement, NIH State-of-the-Science Conference: Preventing Alzheimer's Disease and Cognitive Decline.* Bethesda, MD: NIH Consensus Development Program.

Nelson, Jamie Lindemann, and Hilde Lindemann Nelson. 1997. *Alzheimer's: Answers to Hard Questions for Families.* New York: Doubleday.

Niebuhr, R. 1956. *An Interpretation of Christian Ethics*. New York: Meridian.

Patel, V., and T. Hope. 1993. "Aggressive Behavior in Elderly People with Dementia: A Review." *International Journal of Geriatric Psychiatry* 8:457-472.

Picot, S. J., S. M. Debanne, K. H. Namazi, and M. L. Wykle. 1997. "Religiosity and Perceived Rewards of Black and White Caregivers." *The Gerontologist* 37:89-101.

Post, S. G. 1990. "Severely Demented Elderly People: A Case against Senicide." *Journal of the American Geriatrics Society* 38:715-718.

——. 1995a. "Alzheimer Disease and the 'Then' Self." *Journal of the Kennedy Institute of Ethics* 5 (4): 307-321.

——. 1995b. *The Moral Challenge of Alzheimer Disease*, 1st ed. Baltimore: Johns Hopkins University Press.

——. 1997. "Physician-Assisted Suicide in Alzheimer Disease." *Journal of the American Geriatrics Society* 45:647-651.

——. 1998. "The Fear of Forgetfulness: A Grassroots Approach to Alzheimer Disease Ethics." *Journal of Clinical Ethics* 9 (1): 71-80.

——. 1999. "Future Scenarios for the Prevention and Delay of Alzheimer Disease Onset in High-Risk Groups: An Ethical Perspective." *American Journal of Preventive Medicine* 16:105-110.

——. 2000. *The Moral Challenge of Alzheimer Disease: Ethical Issues from Diagnosis to Dying*, 2nd ed. Baltimore: Johns Hopkins University Press.

——. 2001. "Tube Feeding and Advanced Progressive Dementia." *The Hastings Center Report* 31 (1): 36-42.

——. 2007. "Stumbling on Joy: Not Always a 'Burden' of Care." *Alzheimer's Care Today* 8 (3): 1.

——. 2014. Keynote Address, "Ethics, Dementia and End of Life Care" (2nd Annual Meeting of the Japanese Association for Clinical Ethics, March 2014). Tokyo.

——. 2020. "Autonomy and Respect in Dementia Care" (8th Annual Meeting of the Japanese Association for Clinical Ethics, March 2020). Tokyo.

Post, S. G., and R. H. Binstock, eds. 2004. *The Fountain of Youth: Cultural, Scientific and Ethical Perspectives on a Biomedical Goal*. New York: Oxford University Press.

Post, S. G., L. E. Ng, J. E. Fischel, M. Bennett, L. Bily, L. Chandran, J. Joyce, B. Locicero, K. McGovern, R. I. McKeefrey, J. V. Rodriguez, and M. W. Roess. 2014. "Empathy and Compassionate Patient Care." *Journal of Evaluation in Clinical Practice* 20:872-880. doi:10.1111/jep.12243.

Post, S. G., and P. J. Whitehouse. 1995. "Fairhill Guidelines on the Ethics of the Care of People with Alzheimer's Disease: A Clinician's Summary." *Journal of the American Geriatrics Society* 43 (12): 1423-1429.

———, eds. 1998. *Genetic Testing for Alzheimer Disease: Ethical and Clinical Issues.* Baltimore: Johns Hopkins University Press.

Post, S. G., P. J. Whitehouse, R. H. Binstock, T. D. Bird, S. K. Eckert, L. A. Farrer, L. M. Fleck, A. D. Gaines, E. T. Juengst, H. Karlinsky, S. Miles, T. H. Murray, K. A. Quaid, N. R. Relkin, A. D. Roses, P. H. St. George-Hyslop, G. A. Sachs, B. Steinbock, and E. F. Truschke. 1997. "The Clinical Introduction of Genetic Testing for Alzheimer Disease: An Ethical Perspective." *Journal of the American Medical Association* 277 (10): 832-836.

Reed, P., J. Carson, and Z. Gibb. 2017. "Transcending the Tragedy Discourse of Dementia: An Ethical Imperative for Promoting Selfhood, Meaningful Relationships, and Well-Being." *AMA Journal of Ethics* 19 (7): 693-703. doi:10.1001/journalofethics.2017.19.7.msoc1-1707.

Reifler, B. V., R. S. Henry, K. A. Sherrill, C. H. Ashbury, and J. S. Bodford. 1992. "A National Demonstration Program on Dementia Day Centers and Respite Services: An Interim Report." *Behavior, Health, and Aging* 2 (3):199-206.

Riley, K. P. 1989. "Psychological Interventions in Alzheimer's Disease." In *Memory, Aging and Dementia*, edited by G. C. Gilmore, P. J. Whitehouse, and M. L. Wykle, 199-211. New York: Springer.

Ripich, D., and M. Wykle. 1990. "Developing Health Care Professionals' Communication Skills with Alzheimer's Disease Patients." Paper presented at the annual meeting of the American Society on Aging, San Francisco.

Rohde, K., E. R. Peskind, and M. A. Raskind. 1995. "Suicide in Two Patients with Alzheimer's Disease." *Journal of the American Geriatrics Society* 43:187-189.

Sabat, S. R. 1994. "Excess Disability and Malignant Social Psychology: A Case Study of Alzheimer's Disease." *Journal of Community and Applied Sociology* 4:157-166.

———. 2001. *The Experience of Alzheimer's Disease: Life through a Tangled Veil.* Oxford: Blackwell.

———. 2018. *Alzheimer's Disease & Dementia: What Everyone Needs to Know.* New York: Oxford University Press.

Sabat, S. R., and X. E. Cagigas. 1997. "Extralinguistic Communication Compensates for Loss of Verbal Fluency: A Case Study of Alzheimer's Disease." *Language and Communication* 17:341-351.

Sabat, S. R., and R. Harre. 1994. "The Alzheimer's Disease Sufferer as a Semiotic Subject." *Philosophy, Psychology, and Psychiatry* 1 (3): 145-160.

Salmoirago-Blotcher, E., K. M. Hovey, C. A. Andrews, and S. G. Post. 2019. "Psychological Traits, Heart Rate Variability, and Risk of Coronary Heart Disease in Healthy Aging Women," *Psychosomatic Medicine* 81 (3): 256-264.

Scarmeas, N., J. A. Luchsinger, N. Schupf, A. M. Brickman, S. Cosentino, M. X. Tang, and Y. Stern. 2009. "Physical Activity, Diet, and Risk of Alzheimer Disease." *Journal of the American Medical Association* 302 (6): 627-637.

Schulze, J., R. Mazzola, and F. Hoffman. 2016. "Incidence of Tube Feeding in 7174 Newly Admitted Nursing Home Residents with and without Dementia." *Current Topics in Care* 31 (1): 27-33.

Sifton, C. B. 2004. *Navigating the Alzheimer's Journey: A Compass for Caregiving*, 1st ed. Baltimore: Health Professions Press.

Singer, P. 1993. *Practical Ethics*, 2nd ed. Cambridge: Cambridge University Press.

Smebye, K. L., M. Kirkevold, and K. Engedal. 2012. "How Do Persons with Dementia Participate in Decision Making Related to Health and Daily Care? A Multi-Care Study." *BMC Health Services Research* 12:241.

Smith, A., and J. R. M. Copeland. 1993. "Rementia: Challenging the Limits of Dementia Care." *International Journal of Geriatric Psychiatry* 12:993-1000.

Spanjer, M. 1994. "Mental Suffering as Justification for Euthanasia in the Netherlands." *Lancet* 343:1630.

State of California. 1987. Title 17, *California Code of Regulations*, Section 2572, Chapter 321, Statutes of 1987, amending Section 410 of the Health and Safety Code.

Stubbe, D. E. 2017. "The Health Care Triad: Optimizing Communication in Dementia Care." *Focus* 15 (1): 65-67.

Swinton, J. 2012. *Dementia: Living in the Memories of God*. Grand Rapids, MI: William B. Eerdmans.

Talbot, M. 2011. *The Holographic Universe*. New York: Harper Perennial.

Teichmann, J. 1985. "The Definition of Person." *Philosophy* 60 (232): 175-185.

Teno, J. M., P. I. Gozalo, and S. L. Mitchell. 2012a. "Does Feeding Tube Insertion and Its Timing Improve Survival?" *Journal of the American Geriatrics Society* 60 (10): 1918-1921.

———. 2012b. "Feeding Tubes and the Prevention or Healing of Pressure Ulcers." *Archives of Internal Medicine* 172 (9): 697-701.

Teno, J. M., D. Meltzer, and S. Mitchell. 2014. "The Role of Physician Specialty and Severely Demented Hospitalized Nursing Home Residents' PEG Feeding Tube Insertions." *Health Affairs* 33 (4): 675-682.

Teno, J. M., S. L. Mitchell, and P. I. Gozalo. 2010. "Hospital Characteristics Associated with Feeding Tube Placement in Nursing Home Residents with

Advanced Cognitive Impairment." *Journal of the American Medical Association* 33 (6): 544-550.

Tomlinson, E. 2015. "Assisted Dying in Dementia: A Systematic Review of the International Literature on Attitudes of Health Professionals, Patients, Carers, and the Public, and the Factors Associated with These." *The International Journal of Geriatric Psychiatry* 30:10-20.

US Department of Health and Human Services, Advisory Panel on Alzheimer's Disease. 1991. *Third Report of the Advisory Panel on Alzheimer's Disease.* Washington, DC: US Department of Health and Human Services.

Vanier, J. 1998. *Becoming Human.* Mahwah, NJ: Paulist Press.

Verkerk, M. 2001. "The Care Perspective and Autonomy." *Medical Health Care and Philosophy* 4 (3): 289-294. doi: 10.1023/a:1012048907443.

Visser, F. E., A. P. Aldenkamp, A. C. van Huffelen, M. Kuilman, J. Overweg, and J. van Wijk. 1997. "Prospective Study of the Prevalence of Alzheimer-Type Dementia in Institutionalized Individuals with Down Syndrome." *American Journal on Mental Retardation* 101 (4): 400-412.

Volicer, L., and A. Hurley, eds. 1998. *Hospice Care for Patients with Advanced Progressive Dementia.* New York: Springer.

Whitehouse, Peter J., and Daniel George. 2008. *The Myth of Alzheimer's Disease: What You Aren't Being Told about Today's Most Dreaded Disease.* New York: St. Martin's Press.

Williams, B. 1973. *Problems of the Self.* Cambridge: Cambridge University Press.

Wisniewski, H. M., W. Silverman, and J. Wegiel. 1994. "Ageing, Alzheimer Disease, and Mental Retardation." *Journal of Intellectual Disability Research* 38:233-239.

Wolfensberger, W. 1972. *The Principle of Normalization in Human Services.* Toronto: National Institute on Mental Retardation.

Wright, A. A., B. Zhang, A. Ray, J. W. Mack, E. Trice, T. Balboni, and H. G. Prigerson. 2008. "Associations between End-of-Life Discussions, Patient Mental Health, Medical Care Near Death, and Caregiver Bereavement Adjustment." *Journal of the American Medical Association* 300 (14): 1665-1673.

Wright, L. K. 1993. *Alzheimer's Disease and Marriage: An Intimate Account.* Newbury Park, CA: Sage Publications.

Yu, D., S. T. Cheng, and J. Wang. 2018. "Unravelling Positive Aspects of Caregiving in Dementia: An Integrative Review of Research Literature." *International Journal of Nursing Studies* 79:1-26.

Zagzebski, L. 2001. "The Uniqueness of Persons." *Journal of Religious Ethics* 29 (3): 401-423.

Zapka, J., E. Amella, and G. Magwood. 2014. "Challenges in Efficacy Research: The Case of Feeding Alternatives in Patients with Dementia." *Journal of Advanced Nursing* 70 (9): 2072-2085.

Zigman, W. B., N. Schupf, E. Serson, and W. Silverman. 1995. "Prevalence of Dementia in Adults with and without Down Syndrome." *American Journal of Mental Retardation* 100 (4): 403-412.

acknowledgments

I thank Mike Splaine, founder of Splaine Consulting after more than twenty years as director of advocacy for the Alzheimer's Association Washington offices. Together, Mikey and I developed and conducted ethics workshops across the United States throughout the 1990s. I continue to collaborate in his "live alone" conferences, which are devoted to the care of deeply forgetful people without families to rely on.

I thank Rev. Dr. Jade C. Angelica, a national leader in Alzheimer's care workshops, for her excellent appendix to this book: A Caregiver Resilience Program: Meeting Alzheimer's: Learning to Communicate and Connect, which enjoys a popular following. See Healing Moments for Alzheimer's (www.healingmoments.org) for more information.

I thank the distinguished writer and editor Ann Bradley, who was kind enough to help editorially with the entire manuscript prior to submission. She is a loyal and outstanding editor and I thank Ann for being a true professional.

I gratefully acknowledge Peter J. Whitehouse, MD, PhD, who arrived at Case Western Reserve School of Medicine in 1986 to lead the newly formed Alzheimer's Center. I was privileged to work for Dr. Whitehouse for many years as we developed the center in multiple areas, especially in the social relational aspects of quality of lives, clinical ethics, and policy. Our collaborative "Fairhill Guidelines on Ethics of the Care of People with Alzheimer's Disease: A Clinician's Summary" (*Journal of the*

American Geriatrics Society 43, no. 12 [1995]: 1423-1429) served as the foundation of national ethics guidelines for the Alzheimer's Association both in the United States and across Canada. Dr. Whitehouse and I continue to communicate and collaborate to this day.

In addition, as director of the Center for Medical Humanities, Compassionate Care and Bioethics at the Renaissance School of Medicine at Stony Brook University (2008-present), I thank my many Stony Brook colleagues and students. In particular, I acknowledge the contribution of Phyllis Migdal, MD, MA, to chapter six of this book. I also thank a number of graduate students who helped me wrestle with the questions raised in chapter three. They were part of a spring 2018 graduate course on deeply forgetful people, ethics, and film at the center. These students all contributed a number of clarifications to the chapter which I was

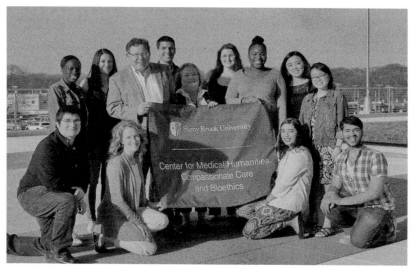

Courtesy of the author

Graduate students in Spring 2018 course on bioethics, film, and the progression of dementia. (*Bottom row kneeling, left to right*) Frank Cordova, Jennifer Kolar, RN, Sara Rahman, Eman Kazi. (*Middle row holding flag, left to right*) Stephen G. Post, PhD, Kathleen Culver, DNP, RN, CPNP, Chelsea Hall. (*Top row, left to right*) Coumba Sy, Alex Wagner, Gregg Cantor, MD, Yakaterina "Kat" Okouneva, Emili Li, Lauren L. Chan.

happy to include. Special thanks to Gregg Cantor, MD, for his helpful updates on novel anti-dementia drugs.

Finally, I must express appreciation to my wife, Mitsuko, and my adult children, Emma and Andrew. There were many nights and weekends for years when I was on the road working with deeply forgetful people and their families or doing clinical ethics consultations in Cleveland or elsewhere around the country, and I did not make it home until late. There were the big trips to faraway places like Sydney and Tokyo that kept me from being fully present at times. I thank them for understanding that I did my best to balance my commitments as a husband and father with my passion to improve the quality of lives of deeply forgetful people and their caregivers.

In essence, this book celebrates the love that caregivers have for deeply forgetful people, and thus I want to acknowledge the support of the John Templeton Foundation and the Institute for Research on Unlimited Love (www.unlimitedloveinstitute.org), for which I have served as founding president since 2001.

Throughout my two decades as a professor at Case Western Reserve School of Medicine I attended St. Paul's Episcopal Church in Cleveland Heights, where I found a community of supportive people who appreciated my work. I would also like to thank St. Paul's School in New Hampshire, where as a young boy I was encouraged to regularly visit the nearby "resting home" on Pleasant Street to play classical guitar for deeply forgetful people.

index